TRADITIONAL FOOD GUIDE

FOR THE ALASKA NATIVE PEOPLE

SECOND EDITION
2015

Written by:

The Alaska Native People

Christine A. DeCourtney, MPA

Desiree M. Jackson, BS, RD, LD

Karen M. Morgan, BA

Nutrition

Elizabeth D. Nobmann, Ph.D, MPH, RD

Melissa A. Chlupach, MS, RD, LD*

Susan Hoyt, MS, RD, LD

Jennifer S. Johnson, MPH, RD

Editing

Marie J. Lavigne, LMSW

Lakota R. Murray, MEd

Judith M. Muller, MHA

Stacy Kelley, MPH*

*Second Edition

1

Where foods are found in Alaska

Each area of Alaska depends on different types of animals, fish and plants. Some examples are...

Low bush salmonberries are gathered in Northern and Western communities

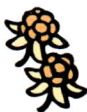

Salmon are harvested in coastal and river communities

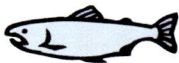

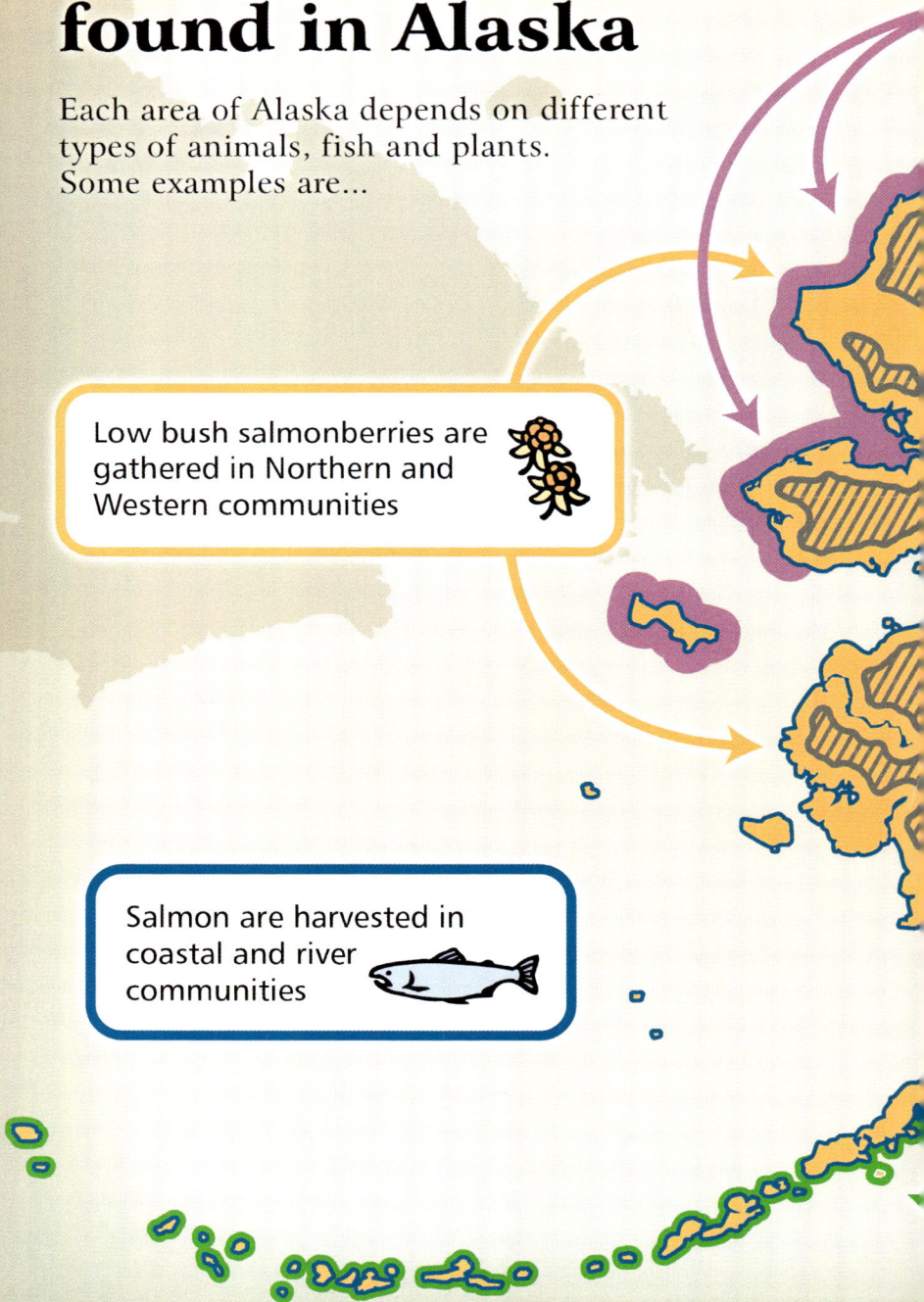

Whales are hunted along the Arctic Coast

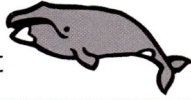

Caribou are hunted in the tundra and forest areas across the state

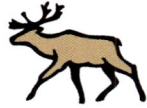

Geese are hunted all over Alaska

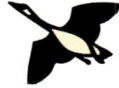

Beach Asparagus is gathered in Southeast, along the Gulf of Alaska and Aleutian Island communities

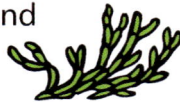

TABLE OF CONTENTS

Food from the Sea (continued)

PLANTS

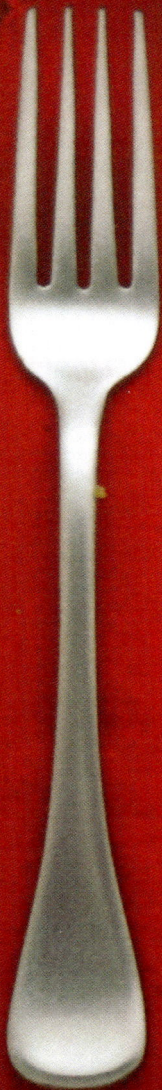
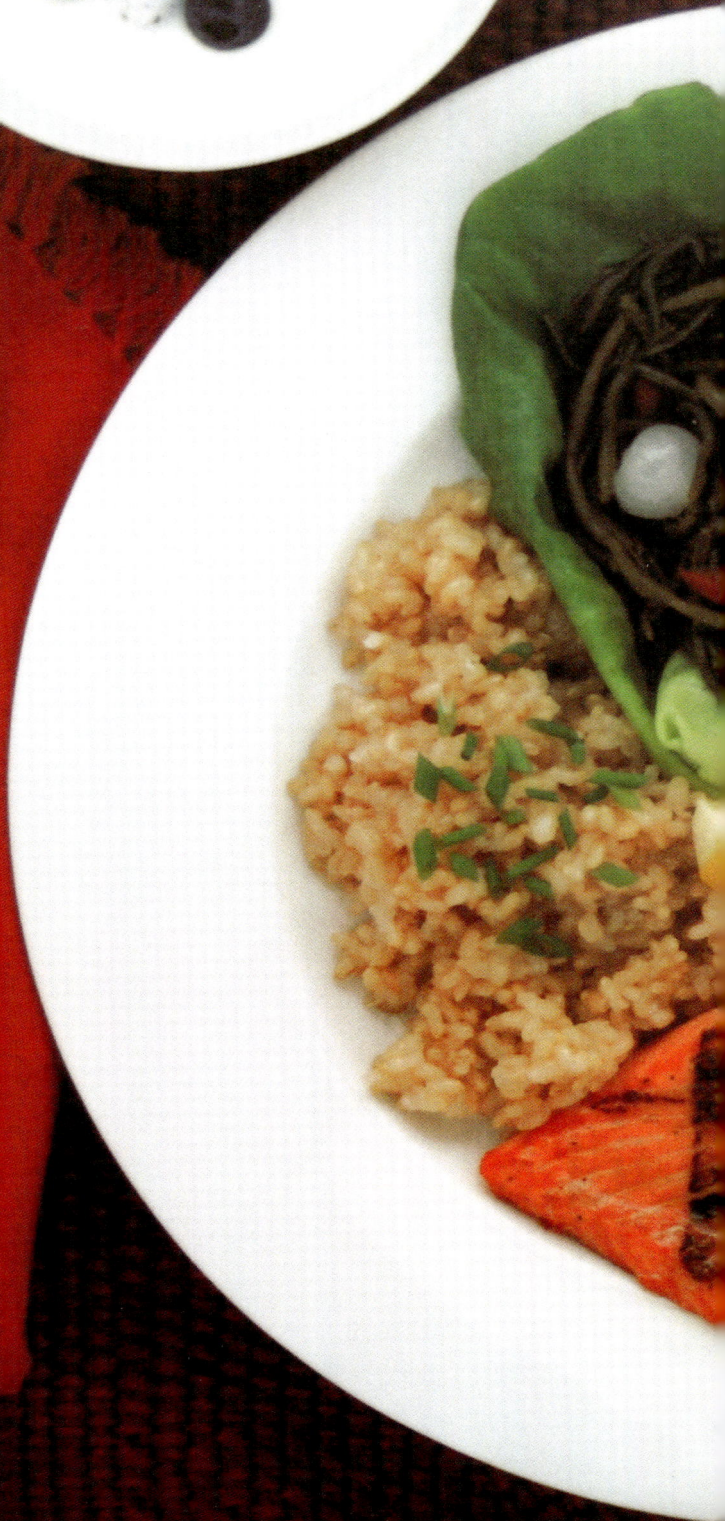
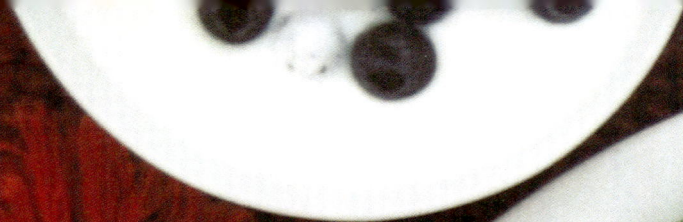

Salmon, Sea Asparagus and Brown Rice

SouthEast Alaska Regional Health Consortium Diabetes Program

9

INTRODUCTION

The first edition of the Traditional Food Guide was designed to support Alaska Native cancer patients who wanted to continue to eat their comforting and nutritious wild foods during treatment. Some healthcare providers were not familiar with the foods and recommended that they not be eaten.

The Traditional Food Guide was far more successful than anticipated. Three printings were sold out and 14,000 copies distributed. Even though the book said "cancer" on the cover, many people bought and used the book. Alaska Native elders were proud to see their foods in the book along with other foods from different parts of Alaska that they did not know about. The book is used by schools, universities, and Community Health Aide Program (CHAP) clinics. Some community tribal councils bought the book for every family. Other health programs, like diabetes, bought the book to share. It was accepted as the only book of its kind and placed in Alaska's National Park book stores after a lengthy approval process.

Pete H. Sovalik Jr. and Belva Patuk Kignak review the Traditional Food Guide   *Roy Corral*

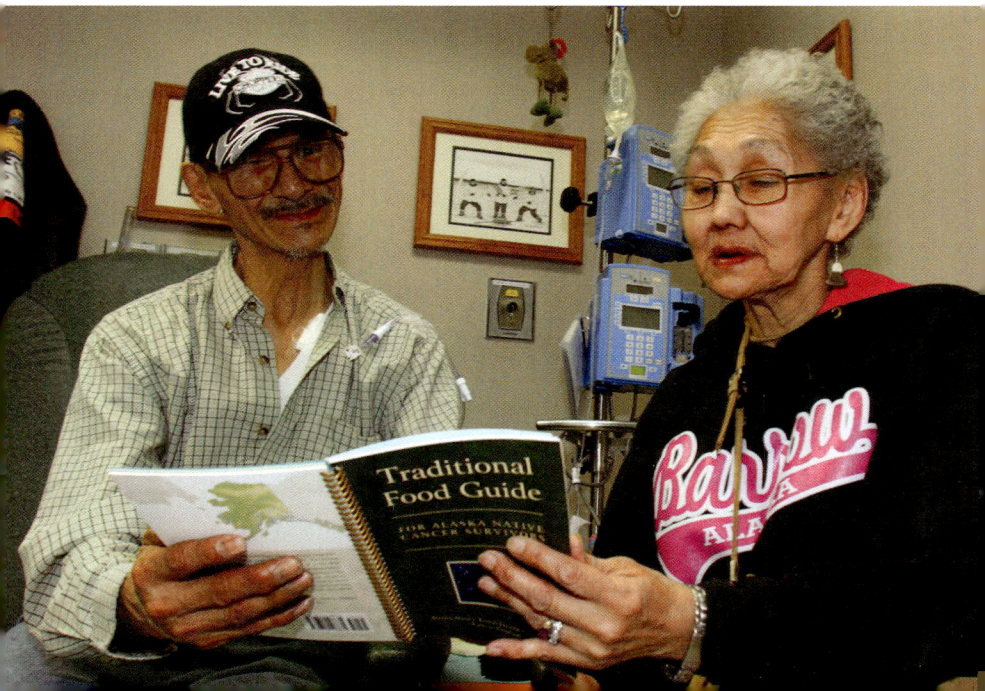

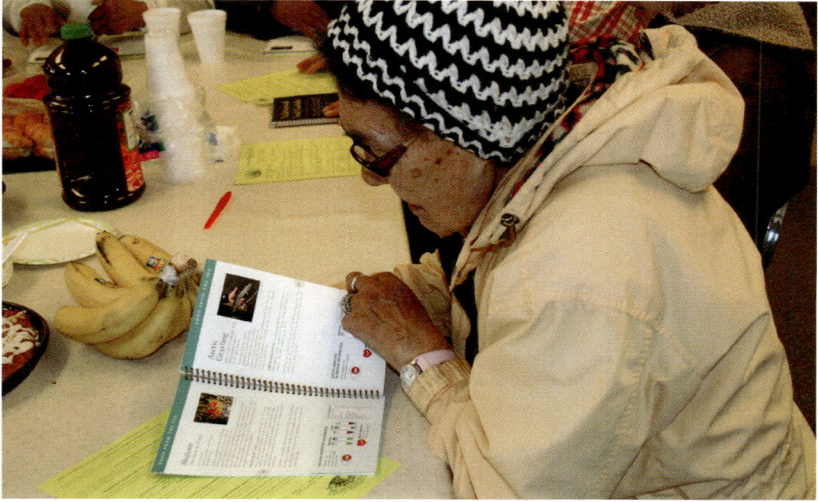

Elder from Kaktovik, AK reading the Traditional Food Guide.

Christine DeCourtney

We have decided to develop a second addition of the book to provide additional information. While the foods and nutrition information remain the same, we have added new material including healthy lifestyle information that was printed in our "Traditional Food Guide Activity Book" distributed annually to schools and other programs for children 8-10 years throughout Alaska. It is now in its fourth printing with over 20,000 copies distributed.

The second edition of the Traditional Food Guide represents different uses by recognizing that the guide is an important tool for healthy living for the youngest child to the oldest elder. It is also a guide to help people with diseases like cancer, diabetes or heart disease learn more about nutrition and eat better foods.

"My husband and son go out every summer, from May to October, in his home town on the lower Yukon and fish, and hunt moose and birds. So my freezer's full at home."

– Ann Lawrence, Anchorage (originally from Mountain Village)

TRADITIONAL FOODS –
Part of a Healthy Lifestyle

Traditional foods are an important part of the Alaska Native culture. The gathering, hunting, preserving and eating of traditional foods is more than just a diet—it's a way of life for Alaska Native people. A subsistence lifestyle has long connected the people with the land and sea through celebrated rituals and practices passed down from generation to generation—from caribou hunting grounds to fish and berry picking camps.

What Alaska Native people eat today is significantly different from what their ancestors ate. The diet includes a combination of traditional and store-bought packaged foods. This contrasts with the diets of the past which relied more heavily on a subsistence lifestyle. Today importance is placed on returning to a traditional lifestyle and diet. The nutritional and physical benefits to this come from eating a diet low in unhealthy fat and cholesterol; eating more animal sources of protein; eating foods without chemicals and additives; and getting more physical activity by gathering, fishing hunting and preserving traditional (wild) Native foods.

What Alaska Native people eat today is significantly different from what their ancestors ate.

While Alaska Native people know the value of their traditional foods, it is only recently that nutritional values of these foods have become available. Previously, there was no food database that contained traditional food information. In the late 1980s, Elizabeth Nobmann, Ph.D, MPH, RD began working to identify nutrient values of traditional foods. In 1992 a nutrient guide for over 160 traditional foods was completed. Without Dr. Nobmann's dedication and pioneer work in supporting the high nutrient value in Alaska's wild foods, this guide would not be possible.

Traditional foods not only provide a nutritional and physical benefit, they also provide comfort. There are special meanings and memories associated with wild and traditional foods. Certain foods used in traditional gatherings provide an opportunity to bring an entire community together to share gathered food.

The food guide includes sections on nutrition, food safety and food sources from the land and sea. The food pages reference the Alaska Native names, history and preparation information and include personal stories. Since there are different names for many traditional Native foods, the guide tries to address the differences by noting the more commonly known names rather than focusing on specific foods from each Alaska region.

REMEMBER—this is your book! Share it with family, friends and your healthcare team. Together we can learn to have a healthier lifestyle.

Note: The Traditional Food Guide provides general nutrition information. It is not meant to substitute for recommendations from your healthcare team. Please check with your healthcare team about your special nutrition needs.

Bristol Bay residents gathering roe on kelp at Metervik Bay   *Fritz Johnson*

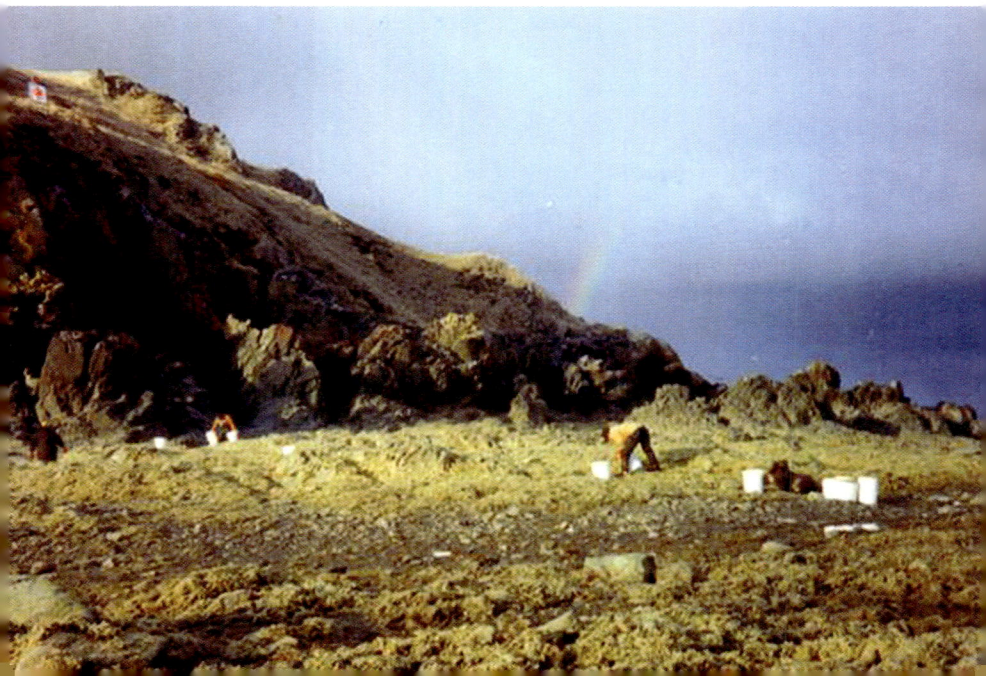

Urban Living & Subsistence Foods

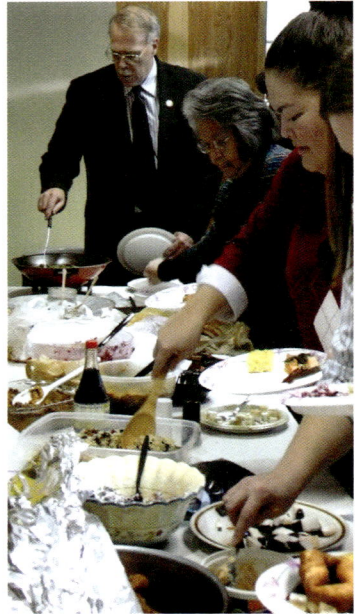

Urban potluck

Nowhere else in the United States is there such a strong reliance on traditional foods and non-food resources gathered from the land and sea as there is in Alaska. Eleven different Alaska Native cultures are spread across more than 200 urban and rural communities. Common ground shared by all of Alaska Native cultures is the importance traditional Native foods have in everyday living.

14

Alaskans living in rural areas harvest about 44 million pounds of wild food each year, an average of about 375 pounds per person. Urban Alaskans harvest about 10 million pounds of wild foods, an average of about 22 pounds per person. The highest amount of wild foods harvested per person occurs within Western and Interior Alaska.

With the mix of wild food available throughout our state, it is no wonder that traditional Native foods are shared through informal trade networks and exchanges between family and friends living in rural Alaska and their extended family living in more urban areas. It is not uncommon to trade a gallon plastic storage bag of salmonberries from the Yukon-Kuskokwim for some caribou or whale meat from the North Slope.

The large distances between family and friends and the desire to taste favorite Native foods from "back home" are commonly bridged through regular Native food gatherings with family, friends, and co-workers. Enjoying our traditional Native foods through sharing is what brings us together and connects us to our past.

Traditional Foods & Social Media

In today's technologically advanced world, social media websites and applications such as Facebook®, Instagram®, and Tumblr® make it easy to virtually share the traditional foods we harvest from the land and sea. We don't give a second thought about "posting" comments and pictures of a tasty, mouthwatering recipe, a care package sent to a loved one living miles away from "back home," or of family and friends gathering to share their treasured traditional foods.

Our virtual sharing lives on after the post and serves as a reminder that sharing is not only done face-to-face, but done easily through social media. We are able to reach our network of family and friends instantly and share what is happening in the present and good memories from the past.

Eskimo Salad by Mellisa Heflin,
Anchorage (originally from Nome, AK)

Made to your liking with seal meat, muktuk, salmon, herring eggs, carrots, onions, willow or beach greens, and drizzled with seal oil. Tastes better when enjoyed with friends and family!

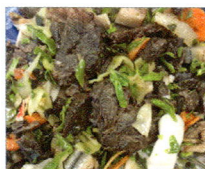

Traditional Foods from "Back Home"
by Vernita Bunyan, Fort Campbell, KY
(originally from Hooper Bay, AK)

Sergeant Vernita Bunyan has been enlisted with the U.S. Army for eight years and is currently stationed at Fort Campbell, Kentucky. When she visits Hooper Bay she usually brings back some of her Native foods. On a recent visit by her sister, she received as she put it, "a ton of food from family members back home. I didn't expect a lot of food to fill the whole freezer. So when I received the food, I ended up throwing out the store bought food in order to stuff my freezer with Eskimo food. I will take my Native food from family any day over store bought food."

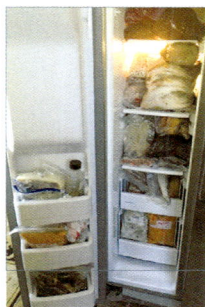

Alaska Native People living in Anchorage talk about their favorite foods.

"I miss whitefish and rhubarb akutaq. My cousins and I would go gather rhubarb and catch whitefish so our Ama (grandmother) would make us akutaq."

– Quentin Simeon, Anchorage (originally from Bethel, Aniak)

" I miss visiting with families at fish camp. Enjoying their company – drinking coffee or tea and eating and visiting. When I am on the river in a boat I feel connected to the land and water – our Athabascan people have been living along the Yukon for centuries. I miss the potlatches for celebrations and memorials."

– Fred Olin, Anchorage (originally from Ruby and Galena)

"Just this weekend we went picking blackberries up on Flattop. While there picking berries, we ran into family I hadn't seen in a long time. We had a wonderful time getting together. It was just like we were back home."

– Laura M. Apatiki, Anchorage (originally from St. Lawrence Island)

16

"I fish and gather my own berries at least once a year. My family and friends bring in Native foods for me once or twice a year... I miss everything about home – poke fish (dry fish soaked in seal oil), dried seal meat, and the fresh fish gathered all summer long (whitefish and salmon). I really miss fresh fish and tundra greens (sourdock)."

– Martha Ray, Anchorage (originally from Hooper Bay)

"[I miss] the ease of access to [subsistence activities back home] the most. When you are at home, the store is your backyard, or just up or down the river. In Anchorage or in urban communities, the best places seem so far away, even if they are not. But [even more], the urban communities make you feel disconnected from the earth."

– Quentin Simeon, Anchorage (originally from Bethel, Aniak)

"I continue to live a subsistence life in the big city. I go salmon fishing every summer. And after that I pick berries, from salmonberries to cranberries until the snow falls."

– Martha Ray, Anchorage (originally from Hooper Bay)

The Traditional Foods Activity Book

The Alaska Native Tribal Health Consortium's Cancer Program developed the Traditional Food Guide Activity Book for Alaska Native youth aged 8 to 10 years to help them make healthy lifestyle choices. Each year, rural school districts are provided the activity book free of charge. Thirty-eight school districts around the state have used the activity book, with more than 20,000 copies distributed. For more information, email cancer@anthc.org.

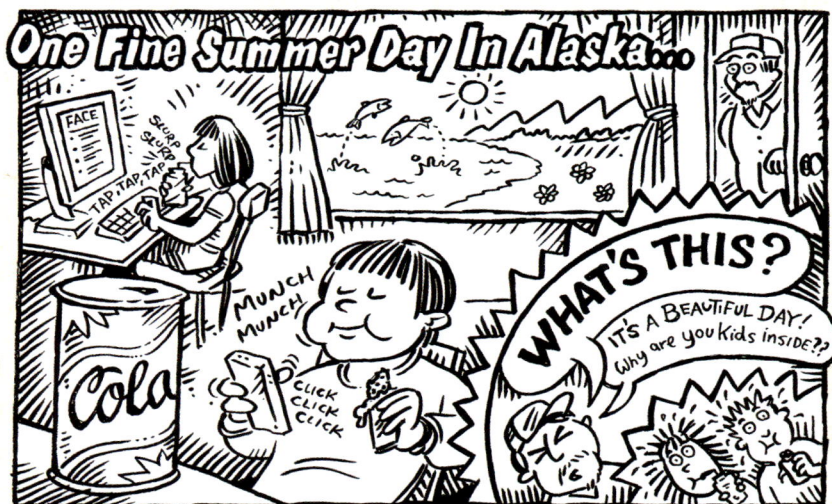

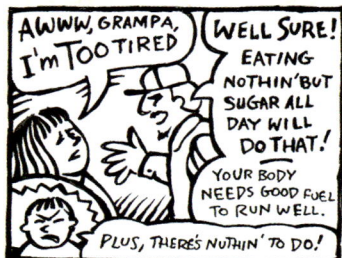

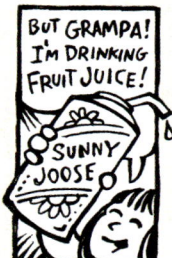

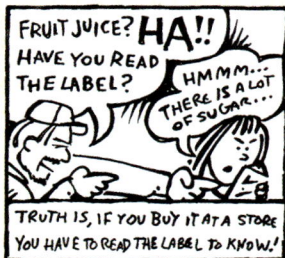

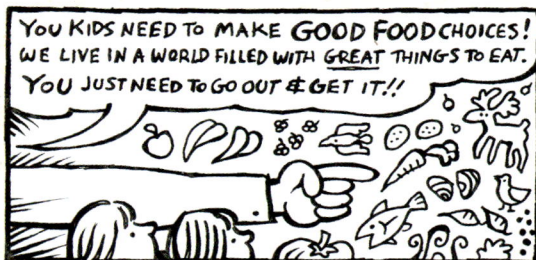

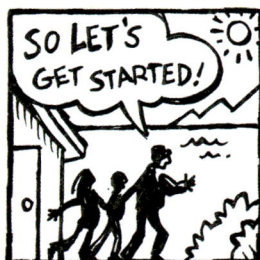

"Thank you for sharing the activity book with my class. The children shared stories about hunting and fishing. The students and staff at our school pick fiddlehead ferns in the spring and other traditional foods." Multi-Grade Teacher, Charter School

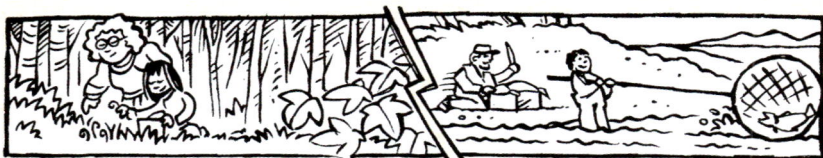

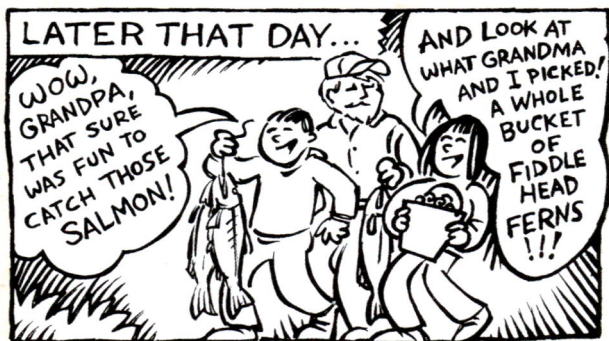

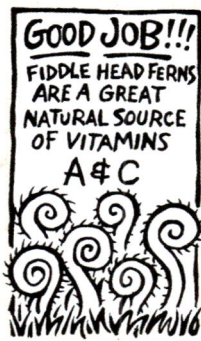

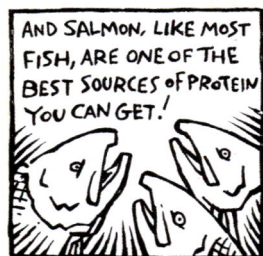

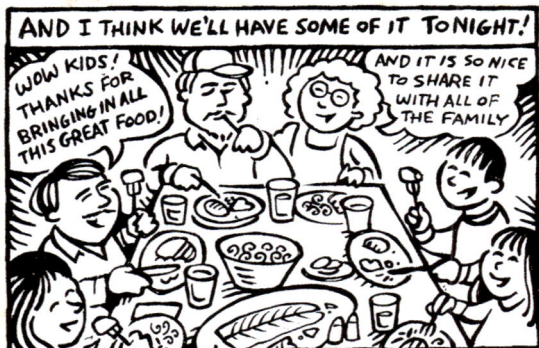

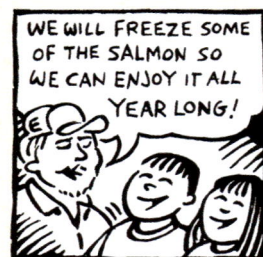

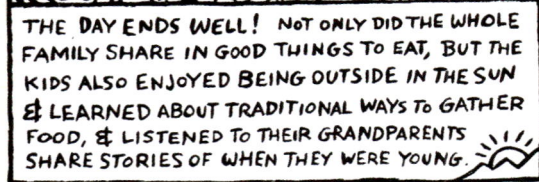

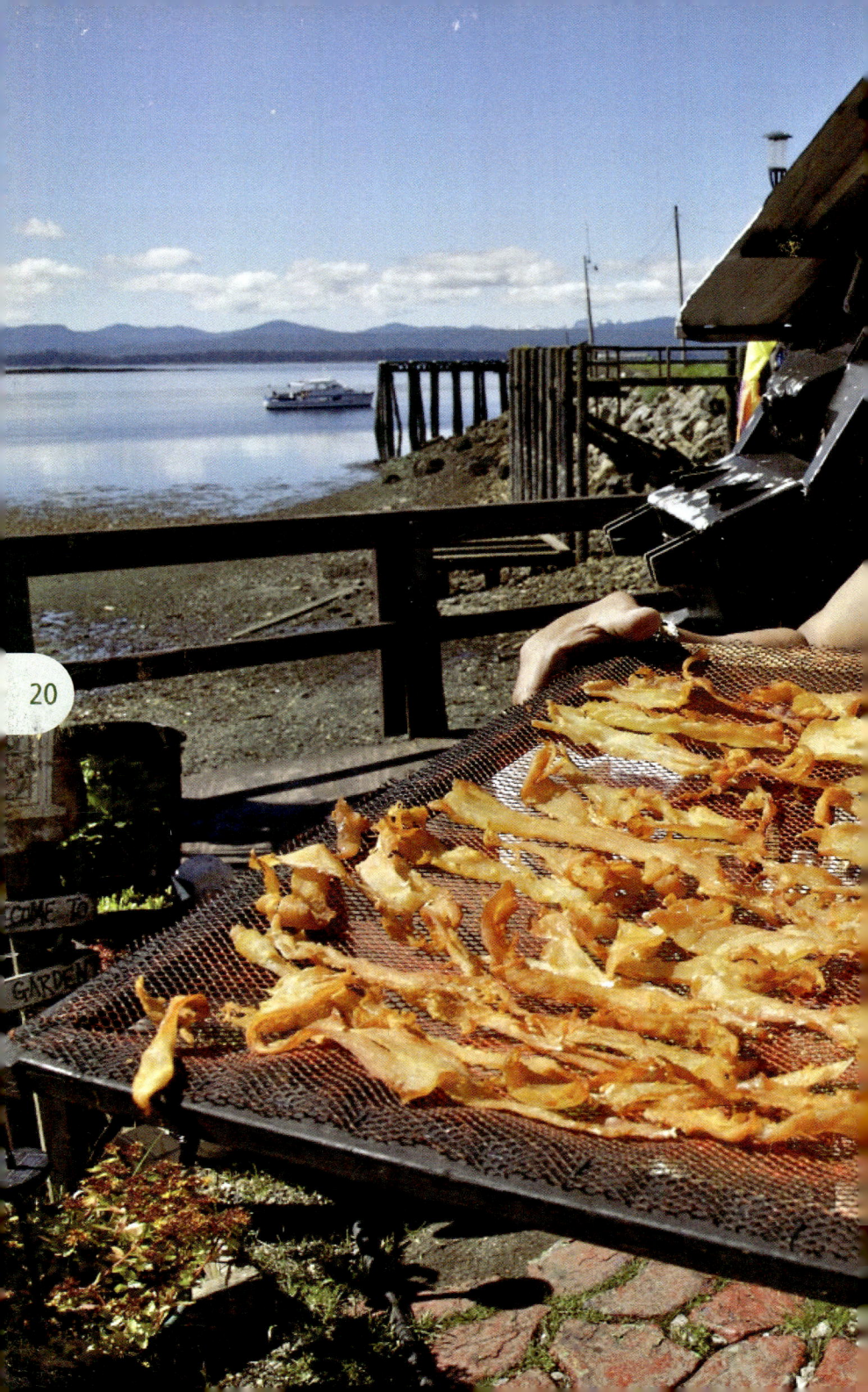

David K. James from Kake, AK holding his smoked halibut

Clark James Mishler

21

TRADITIONAL FOODS: GOOD FOR LIFE

Alaska Native people have been nourished by foods from the land and water for thousands of years. Alaska Native elders pass on ways to harvest and preserve these foods to the next generation. Their lives depended on this information. Each region of Alaska relies on different types of animals, fish and plants to provide nutrients needed to live in a harsh environment.

Traditional foods have a lifelong association to those who eat them. There is a tradition of respect for these foods. This association and respect flows from the gathering or hunting, to the preparation for eating and storing food. Traditionally, Alaska Native people thank the animals who give themselves to be harvested.

Native foods are especially good sources of nutrients like protein, iron and Vitamin A and are low in saturated fat and sugar.

When Alaska Native people hunt, fish, and gather food from the land, there are many benefits. Food is the heart of Alaska Native culture and health. Food provides close ties to the land and the environment and helps keep our traditions alive. Participating in harvesting, preparing, sharing and eating of the foods along with others contributes to our spiritual well being.

"Without ritual, without story-telling, without the drum, without dance, subsistence is only food." – Andrew Paukan

It's difficult in these times to think that we can completely go back to a subsistence lifestyle, with all the modern conveniences and foods available at the local store. However, it is realistic to educate ourselves on the many benefits of traditional foods and learn how to make healthier food choices.

"My mom is 90 years old. It's like she is in her 60's and 70's from eating Native foods."

– Source unknown

People take great comfort from eating Native foods. This guide is meant to show you that the foods you have grown up with are good for your health. The foods in this guide can be used while undergoing cancer treatment, and throughout the recovery and healing process. They are rich in nutrients and healthy for all people. These foods are especially comforting to eat in times of illness and healing.

GATHERING & EATING TRADITIONAL FOODS:

- Contributes to physical fitness and good health
- Keeps people in tune with nature
- Upholds respect for animal and human life
- Encourages sharing in the community
- Is an important part of culture
- Contributes to children's education
- Teaches survival skills
- Provides skills in food preservation and preparation

Note: Plant names may vary among regions. In this guide, we have included all the names that we know.

23

"I think Native foods make people happier."

– Elder

FOOD CHOICES FOR SPECIAL DIETARY NEEDS

Ways to increase protein:

- Eat fish as part of your meals or as a snack
- Eat moose, caribou, seal and other meats
- Eat dried meat or fish
- Add one cup of non-fat dry milk to 1 quart whole milk (4 cups to 1 gallon), use in cooking, hot cereals and shakes
- Eat yogurt or cottage cheese with fruit
- Eat wild bird eggs and store-bought eggs
- Eat peanut butter, beans, nuts, tofu and seeds

FIBER IS AN IMPORTANT PART OF FOOD CHOICES

Eating fiber can:

- Help lower bad cholesterol
- Help lower high blood pressure
- Help protect against heart disease
- Clean out the intestines of waste
- Help you feel full
- Help protect against gall bladder disease, colon cancer, and hemorrhoids
- Help prevent constipation

Simple ways to get more fiber in your diet:

- Eat blueberries or salmonberries, or any berries fresh or frozen
- Gather and eat sourdock and other Alaska wild greens
- Eat whole fruit, dried or canned fruit instead of juice
- Have oatmeal or mush for breakfast
- Add barley or brown rice to soup
- Add beans or peas to soups or tacos

- Have baked beans or split pea soup
- Eat whole wheat bread instead of white bread
- Try substituting whole wheat flour for some of the white flour in baking

IDEAS TO HELP MANAGE BEING TIRED

A healthy diet and exercise may help reduce being tired that may be part of having cancer, heart disease, diabetes or other diseases. Check with your healthcare team!

Ways to reduce being tired:

- Eat more protein
- Don't skip meals, especially breakfast
- Try 3 medium-sized meals and 2 healthy snacks
- Avoid sugar and simple sugar products like candy
- Eat plenty of calories
- Drink lots of water, milk, fruit and vegetable juice
- Exercise—even for 10 minutes a day

INCREASING APPETITE

Tips for increasing appetite:

- Eat when you feel well or when you feel hungry
- Surround yourself with good smells, such as the smell of freshly baked bread
- Eat with friends and family
- Eat smaller meals frequently and have snacks between meals
- Brush your teeth, or wipe the inside of your mouth with a wash cloth and rinse
- Eat foods you really like when your appetite is not good
- Give food a chance; remember that what sounds bad today may sound good tomorrow

INCREASING CALORIES

Sometimes losing weight is important to leading a healthy lifestyle. But in other situations, too much weight loss can make you feel very tired. Check with your healthcare team!

Here are some tips to add calories:

- Add more calories to a meal by adding butter, cheese, seal oil, muktuk, walrus blubber, fish, yogurt or ice-cream.

- Add seal oil to foods like dried fish, vegetables or soup.

- Eat akutaq with fat and berries

- Eat fatty fish like salmon

- Add butter to potatoes, hot cereal, rice, noodles, and cooked vegetables

- Use mayonnaise and salad dressing

- Have a bedtime snack like hot chocolate or hot Tang, tea and crackers with butter and jelly.

- Try salty not sweet foods, dry foods like dry toast, or ginger ale, tea, popsicles and clear liquids like broth.

- If swallowing is difficult, mash foods or add gravies.

Note: If you are experiencing weight loss, talk to your healthcare team.

HEALTHY LIFESTYLE

In general, a healthy diet is a healing diet. Maintaining a healthy weight is an important part of a healthy lifestyle. Ask your healthcare team what a healthy weight is for you.

Maintaining a healthy weight:

- Drink plenty of water.

- Reduce the amount of fat and sugar you eat.

- Recognize and be aware of when and why you eat

- Eat breakfast

- Eat more traditional foods, complex carbohydrates (pasta, rice) and high fiber foods (whole grain bread and cereals, beans).

- Eat more fruits and vegetables

- Use less fat when cooking: boil, broil, bake, steam, grill and microwave your foods
- Avoid soda and other sugary beverages like Kool-Aid and Tang

PHYSICAL ACTIVITY

Maintaining or increasing fitness can improve your quality of life, including being able to pick more berries, play with children or grandchildren or catching more fish. Exercise does not have to be hard or cause discomfort. It can be broken up into small amounts of time over a day.

Physical activity:

- Keeps the heart in shape
- Burns off calories from the food you eat
- Improves sleep
- Improves the health of our bodies:
  - Relieves tension and stress
  - Keeps bones strong
  - Improves digestion (helps you avoid constipation)
  - Improves circulation of blood
  - Gives you more energy
  - Generally makes you feel better

Tips to increase physical activity:

- Start slow
- Walk instead of riding in a car, on a four wheeler or on a snow machine
- Ride a bicycle
- Take the stairs instead of the elevator
- Get up and move while watching TV
- Collect and prepare traditional foods
- Aim for 30 minutes of exercise a day

Note: Check with your healthcare team before starting an exercise program.

FOOD NUTRIENTS

To live, we need energy from three sources:

● **PROTEIN**   ● **FAT**   ● **CARBOHYDRATES**

PROTEIN helps build organs and muscles. It helps cells grow and heal. During cancer treatment, healing and recovery, your body may need more protein. Protein is found in many foods. Good sources are caribou, moose and seal, all types of fish, and beans.

FAT supports the body's internal organs and insulates them. It is essential for the function of the nervous system including the brain. No more than 30% of your total daily calories should come from fat. The fat found in traditional Alaska Native foods, like seal oil, salmon, and whale blubber, is rich in heart healthy Omega-3 fatty acids. The fat found in foods from the store, like whole milk, cheese, beef, chicken skin, lard, and butter, contain more unhealthy saturated fat than traditional foods. Saturated fat raises blood cholesterol levels, and is linked to heart disease.

CARBOHYDRATES are the main source of fuel for the muscles and brain, and are the favorite source of fuel for every cell in your body. There are two types of carbohydrates: complex and simple sugars. Complex carbohydrates tend to be healthier and more satisfying, and an excellent source of vitamins and minerals. Examples include rice, beans, oatmeal, seaweed and berries.

Simple sugars break down rapidly. Foods with simple sugars may be less nutritious than complex carbohydrates. Examples are jam, jelly, honey, sugar, soda, corn syrup and candy.

"Eat your carrots", the teacher said to the little boy. "They will help you see the moose in the dark." — *Togiak Teacher*

We need many other nutrients from our food:

- **FIBER** • **VITAMIN C** • **VITAMIN A**
- **IRON** • **CALCIUM**

FIBER is used by the body to clean out the intestinal tract – it helps the bowels to move. It cannot be digested and has no calories. Fiber is found in vegetables and fruits including Alaska wild greens and berries. It is also found in beans and whole grains like whole wheat bread, brown rice, and whole grain cereal including oatmeal. Be sure to drink lots of water when eating fiber-rich foods.

We need **VITAMINS & MINERALS** from food every day. Vitamins and minerals play a key role in all of the body's functions. You may get them from food or take a supplement. The body uses different vitamins for different functions.

VITAMIN C is used by your body's immune system to fight infection. Vitamin C is also important for healthy teeth, gums and blood vessels. Vitamin C helps the body use iron from food. Berries are a good Vitamin C food source as well as oranges, grapefruit, and 100% fruit juices. One benefit of getting Vitamin C from foods rather than supplements or fortified foods (example: Tang) is that Vitamin C rich foods provide other healthy nutrients your body needs.

"Every summer we went to berry camp for 1-2 weeks. When the tide came in, we left for camp in our boat loaded with supplies. We got to camp just as the sun was setting. My father, Dick Bunyan, put out a net to catch fish for dinner. We picked berries all day and filled 3 different sized barrels. I miss the tundra—way out there away from the village, city and road noise. I miss the fresh air, the quietness and the birds singing… and the berries."

– Patricia Bunyan, Anchorage (originally from Hooper Bay)

VITAMIN A is important for vision – especially night vision. It is also used to keep skin healthy, and contributes to a strong immune system. Good sources of Vitamin A are local berries, marine mammal oil (seal or whale), and liver. Beta-carotene is a form of Vitamin A found in highbush salmonberries, carrots, pumpkin, apricots, collard greens, kale, sweet potatoes, parsley, and spinach. It is best to get your Vitamin A from food, because Vitamin A can build up to toxic levels in the body when large amounts are taken by supplement.

IRON helps the body build muscles and blood which carries oxygen through your bloodstream helping you to be alert and to think clearly. Your body requires more iron when you are growing. Rich sources include meat from seal and whale, meat from moose and caribou, liver and other organ meats. The level of iron in these meats is much higher than in meats from the store. Plant sources of iron include seaweed, dried fruits, whole grains, beans and leafy green vegetables.

CALCIUM is the most abundant mineral in the human body, making up about 2% of total body weight. 99% of the body's calcium is in bones and teeth. The other 1% helps the heart beat correctly, nerves function, blood to clot, and helps break down food and use the energy. Alaskans get calcium from eating whole fish, including the skin and bones such as canned fish with soft bones, and from wild bird eggs with embryos, and seaweed. Dairy products like milk and cheese are sources of calcium, along with orange juice or soy milk fortified with calcium, green leafy vegetables, nuts and seeds.

"Happiness is healing. Elders need to taste the food they've grown up on so they can feel good about themselves again – it's a healing thing." -Frank Wright, Hoonah

DAILY FOOD GUIDE

To get these nutrients follow this Daily Food Guide:

GRAIN PRODUCTS:
6 to 8 servings a day

VEGETABLES & FRUITS:
6 to 10 servings a day

MILK PRODUCTS & SUBSTITUTES:
2 to 4 servings a day

MEATS, FISH, EGGS & BEANS:
2 to 3 servings a day

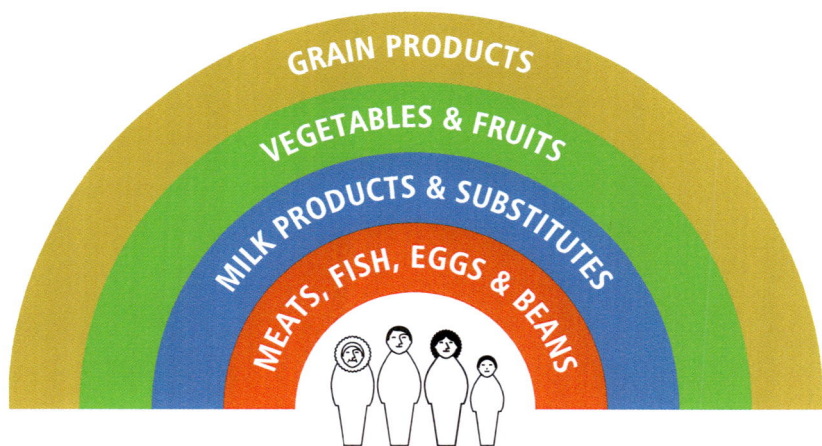

GRAIN PRODUCTS

VEGETABLES & FRUITS

MILK PRODUCTS & SUBSTITUTES

MEATS, FISH, EGGS & BEANS

Healthy eating plus physical activity equals a healthy lifestyle.

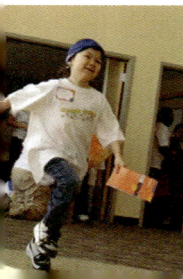

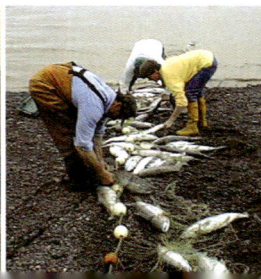

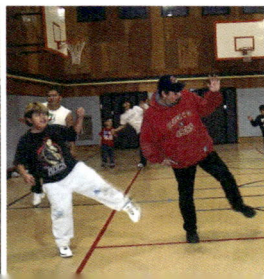

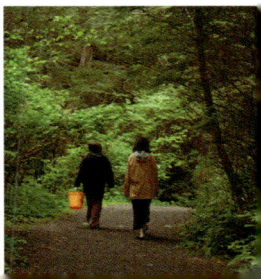

Your Visual Guide to Healthier Eating

The Plate Method: Lunch and Dinner

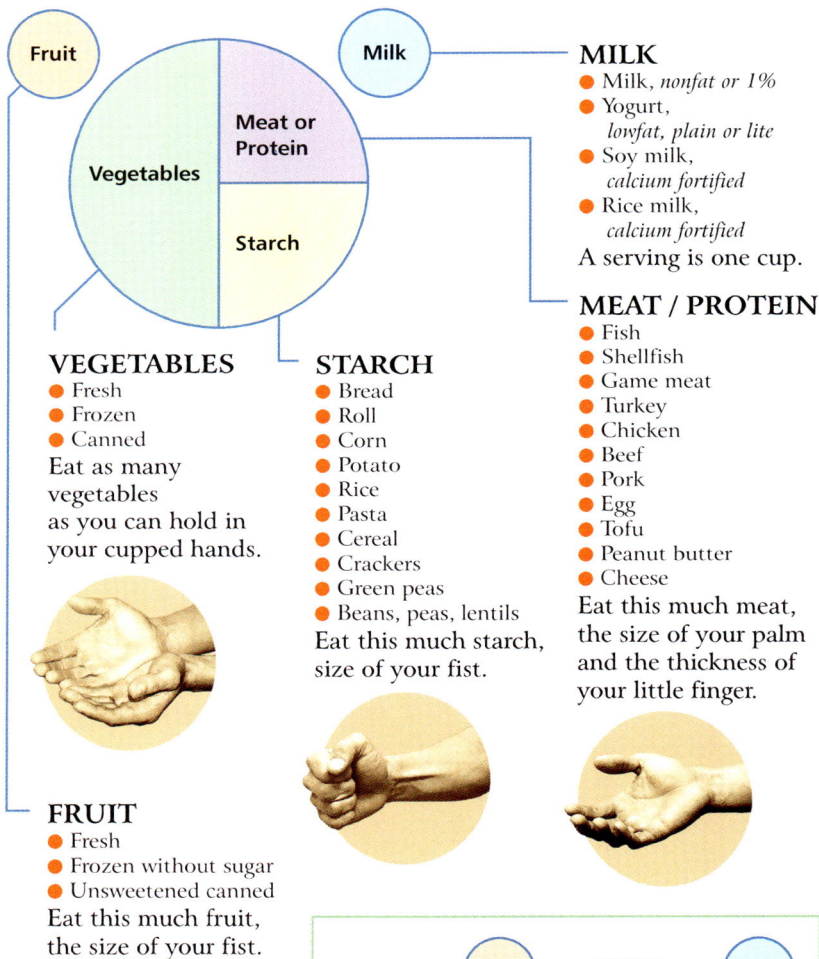

Fruit

Milk

Meat or Protein

Vegetables

Starch

MILK
- Milk, *nonfat or 1%*
- Yogurt, *lowfat, plain or lite*
- Soy milk, *calcium fortified*
- Rice milk, *calcium fortified*

A serving is one cup.

MEAT / PROTEIN
- Fish
- Shellfish
- Game meat
- Turkey
- Chicken
- Beef
- Pork
- Egg
- Tofu
- Peanut butter
- Cheese

Eat this much meat, the size of your palm and the thickness of your little finger.

VEGETABLES
- Fresh
- Frozen
- Canned

Eat as many vegetables as you can hold in your cupped hands.

STARCH
- Bread
- Roll
- Corn
- Potato
- Rice
- Pasta
- Cereal
- Crackers
- Green peas
- Beans, peas, lentils

Eat this much starch, size of your fist.

FRUIT
- Fresh
- Frozen without sugar
- Unsweetened canned

Eat this much fruit, the size of your fist.

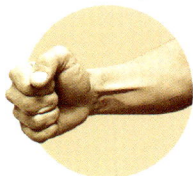

The Plate Method: Breakfast

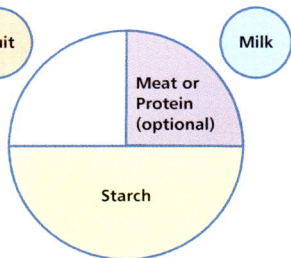

Fruit

Milk

Meat or Protein (optional)

Starch

Adapted from SouthEast Alaska Regional Health Consortium Diabetes Program

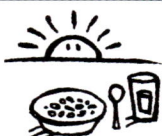

MORNING • • • • • • • • • • **NOON** • • • • • • • • • • **EVENING** • • • • • • • •

Breakfast
The most important meal of the day

Snack
A fruit or vegetable to carry you through to lunch

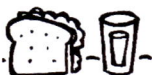

Lunch
A meal rich with protein and carbs

Snack
Have a couple of salmon strips or other healthy snack

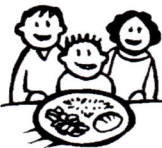

Dinner
Best with the whole family

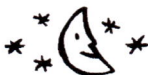

Have a Good Night!

When to Eat

- **Eat breakfast every day** – it gives you energy that you need to start the day and do well at work and in school!

- **Don't skip meals** – including breakfast, lunch and dinner

- **Make sure your lunch has protein** (peanut butter sandwich, salmon) so you don't have a 3 o'clock "crash"

- **Chew food slowly** – enjoy each bite!

- **Drink water** or low- or non-fat milk with each meal

- **Eat before you get too hungry and stop eating when you feel full**

Good snack ideas:

- 1 slice 100% whole-grain bread with peanut butter and blueberry jam

- Snack-size box of raisins

- 6 oz. low-fat yogurt and blueberries

- Small apple or carrots

- A banana, or a small handful of nuts

- Dried salmon strips, caribou or moose jerky

33

Eating before & after physical activity:

- Eat 30-60 minutes before an activity for energy and strength

- Eat within 15 to 60 minutes after an activity to replace muscle fuel

- Drink water before, during, and after physical activity to replace water lost through sweat and prevent dehydration

Understanding the Nutrition Facts

Nutrition food label information on store-bought foods is easier to understand once you know how to "crack the code"!

❶ Start with serving size
Know the amount of food you need for one serving so that you don't eat too much.

❷ Then check calories
Know how much of your daily energy is in one serving.

❸ Limit these nutrients
Watch out for foods with high percentage of saturated and trans fat, sodium, cholesterol, and sugar.

❹ Get enough of these nutrients
Look for foods with high fiber, vitamins and minerals, protein and carbohydrates (other than sugar)

Nutrition Facts
Serving Size: 1 Cup (227g)
Servings Per Container about 4

Amount Per Serving:		
Calories 130	Calories From Fat 0	
		% Daily Value*
Total Fat 0g		**0%**
Saturated Fat 0g		**0%**
Trans Fat 0g		
Cholesterol 0mg		**0%**
Sodium 85mg		**4%**
Total Carbohydrate 9g		**3%**
Dietary Fiber 0g		**0%**
Sugars 9g		
Protein 23g		**46%**
Vitamin A 0%	• Vitamin C 0%	
Calcium 25%	• Iron 0%	

*Percent Daily Values are based on a 2,000 calorie diet. Your daily values may be higher or lower depending on your calorie needs.

INGREDIENTS: GRADE A PASTEURIZED SKIMMED MILK, LIVE YOGURT CULTURES (L. BULGARICUS, S. THERMOPHILUS, L. ACIDOPHILUS, BIFIDUS, L. CASEI)

GRAMS are a unit of measurement that you will find used for food amounts on nutrition labels.
1 OUNCE = 28 GRAMS

Understanding the Ingredients List

Ingredients are listed in order of weight or how much each ingredient is in the food from most to least amount. For example, yogurt is made mostly from milk, so milk is the first ingredient listed.

Compare the differences in ingredients for these two store-bought foods:

CANNED SOCKEYE SALMON: sockeye salmon and salt

CHEETOS: Enriched Corn Meal (Corn Meal, Ferrous Sulfate, Niacin, Thiamin Monoitrate, Riboflavin, and Frolic Acid), Vegetable Oil (corn, canola, soybean, and/or sunflower oil), Cheese Seasoning (Whey, and less than 2% of the Following: Cheddar Cheese, (Cultured Milk, Cheese cultures, Salt, Enzymes). Partially Hydrogenated Soybean Oil, Canola Oil, Maltodextrin, Disodium Phosphate, Sour Cream (Cultured Cream, Nonfat Milk), Artificial Flavor, Monosodium Glutmate, Lactic Acid, Artificial Colors (Including Yellow 6), and Citric Acid. Contains Milk Ingredients.

How to Read the Nutrition Section of This Guide

Each page offers five ways to help you understand the food's nutrition.

1 **Words** - tell nutritional needs for elders, men, women and the percent that one portion of the food provides

2 **Portion size** - the serving of meat and fish that fits in the palm of your hand or is the size of a deck of cards; vegetables, soup and other foods that fit in a cup; and a spoon to show 1 tablespoon for fats and oils.

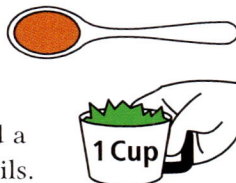

1 Cup

3 **People** - one serving of food meets part of the recommended daily intake of a nutrient that may be different for elders, men, women. Sometimes one food portion meets more than the daily requirements of a nutrient. This is shown by + on the person

4 **Happy Heart** - foods that are good for your heart, low in saturated fat and salt.

5 **Food label** - information that shows standard nutrient values that can be used to compare Native foods to labels on Western foods.

---

1 **BEAVER NUTRITION INFORMATION**

Beaver is an excellent source of protein & iron

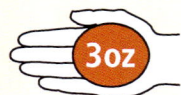

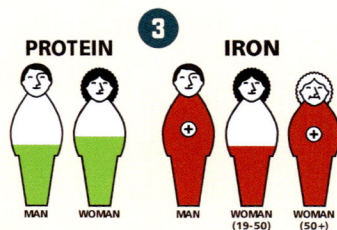

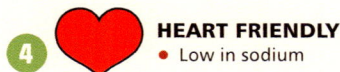

2 3oz

3 PROTEIN   IRON

MAN   WOMAN   MAN   WOMAN (19-50)   WOMAN (50+)

4 HEART FRIENDLY
• Low in sodium

NUTRITION INFORMATION	
Per serving - 3 oz: roasted	
Calories	180
Protein	30 g
Carbohydrate	0 g
Fat	6 g
Calories from fat	30 %
Saturated	2 g
Dietary Fiber	0 g
Cholesterol	99 mg
Sodium	50 mg
Vitamin A	0
Vitamin C	3 mg
Iron	9 mg

"My grandfather and uncle taught me how to hunt
starting when I was 7 years old... I remember sitting in
blinds for hours trying to call ducks and waiting and
waiting. I learned a great deal about patience.
The first ducks were shared with my grandparents, then
my parents and if we had more ducks – the village.
I wouldn't change growing up in White Mountain
and living a subsistence lifestyle.

– Matthew Ione, Anchorage (White Mountain)

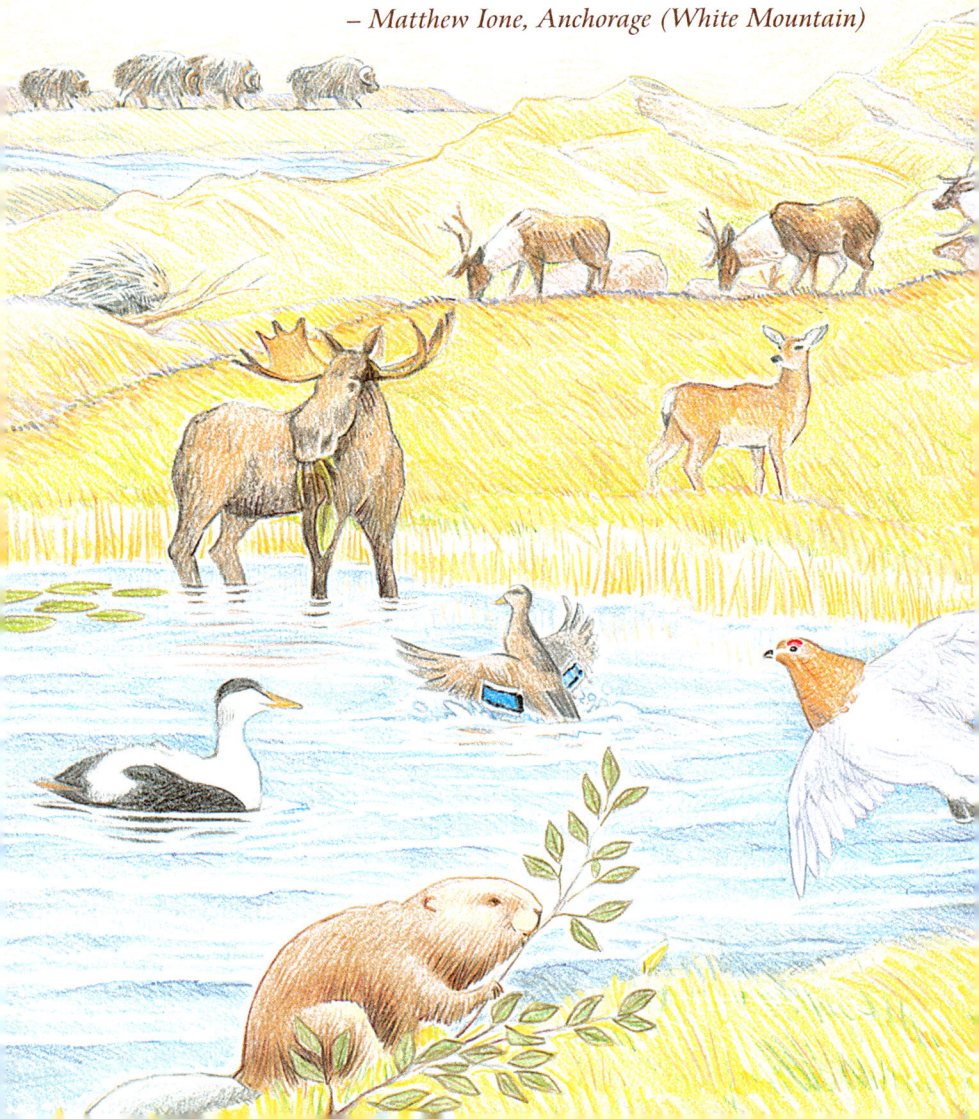

Food from the Land

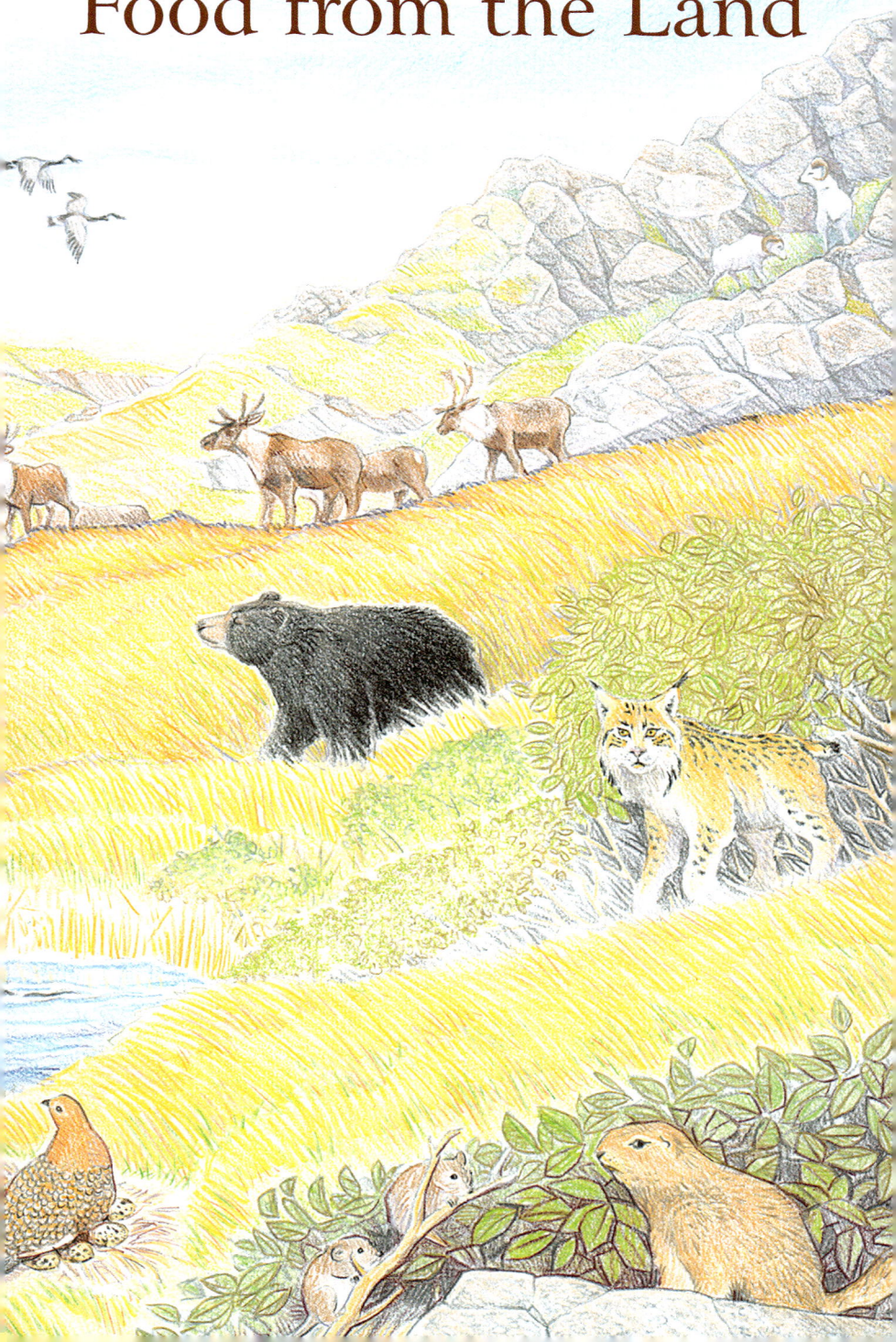

Beaver

NATIVE NAMES: Paluqtaq *(Yup'ik)*,
K'enuy'a *(Dena'ina)*, S'igeidí *(Tlingit)*,
Pajuqtaq *(Iñupiaq)*

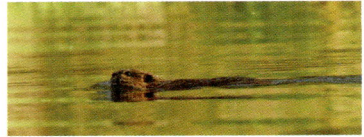

U.S. Fish & Wildlife Service

Beaver can be found throughout the forested regions of the state. Beavers require 2 to 3 feet of water in order to protect themselves from enemies. In areas where the water level is too low, they construct dams along waterways to flood the surrounding area. The pelts of beaver are prized items used to make cold weather items such as coats, hats, and mittens. The meat is prized for the taste and fermented beaver tail is a delicacy.

PREPARATION: Beaver can be roasted, fried, boiled, dried or fermented. Its meat is dark red, fine grained, moist and tender, and when properly prepared, it can taste like pork.

Wolves and beavers were difficult to catch before European contact. Because of the difficulty in obtaining their pelts, the Yup'ik believed these animals must be honored. The Yup'ik people honored wolves and beavers by incorporating their pelts into ceremonial headdress, demonstrating respect to the animal spirits.

"Beaver tail is excellent! We have it at potlatches. When I go home, I can't get enough of it. Its texture is chewy, rubbery, with a good taste, and it is softer than moose nose. To prepare, boil, cool, and peel off the skin after boiling."

– Audrey Armstrong, Huslia

38

BEAVER NUTRITION INFORMATION

Beaver is an excellent source of protein & iron

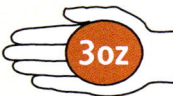

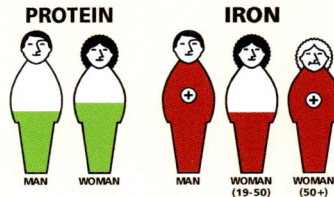

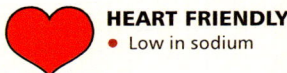

3oz

PROTEIN

MAN   WOMAN

IRON

MAN   WOMAN   WOMAN
     (19-50) (50+)

HEART FRIENDLY
• Low in sodium

NUTRITION INFORMATION	
Per serving - 3 oz: roasted	
Calories	180
Protein	30 g
Carbohydrate	0 g
Fat	6 g
Calories from fat	30 %
Saturated fat	2 g
Dietary Fiber	0 g
Cholesterol	99 mg
Sodium	50 mg
Vitamin A	0
Vitamin C	3 mg
Iron	9 mg

Bone Marrow

NATIVE NAMES: **Pateq** *(Yup'ik),*
K'eyiha *(Dena'ina),*
S'aak s'aak tu.eexí *(Tlingit)*
Tumtux̂ *(Unangam Tunuu),*
Patiq *(Iñupiaq)*

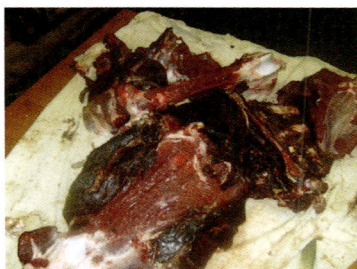
Desiree Jackson

Traditionally, bone marrow was eaten raw, or added to soups and stews. The bone marrow of moose and caribou is a valuable and important part of game animals. Caribou bone marrow is high in healthy fats and rich in iron.

PREPARATION: Bone marrow soup is the most common method of preparing the caribou marrow. Use bones with a lot of marrow (leg bones) with meat left on them. Cut the bones into sections, and when the marrow is heated, it becomes slippery and soft, and it slips right out.

People who had seal oil dipped the cooked meat in the seal oil. The dried meat was kept and wrapped in the fall caribou skin. We also cracked the end bones of the caribou and boiled them until the marrow and the fat settled on top. These were then put into the stomach container, and when we wanted something to mix with our food, we used this marrow and fat.
— *www.alaskool.org*

"*The end of the month, I'm going to Clarks Point. My friends are cooking me buttuk bones and seal oil. That's boiled moose marrow with meat on it to dip in seal oil, with rice on the side. MMMMM....*"
— *Nina Heavener, Clarks Point*

39

BONE MARROW NUTRITION INFORMATION

NUTRITION INFORMATION	
Per serving - 1 oz: cooked	
Calories	222
Protein	2 g
Carbohydrate	0 g
Fat	24 g
Calories from fat	97 %
Saturated fat	NT*
Dietary Fiber	NT*
Cholesterol	NT*
Sodium	NT*
Vitamin A	68 IU
Vitamin C	NT*
Iron	1 mg

*Not Tested

The caribou, Sitka black-tailed deer, and reindeer are members of the deer family and have similar characteristics and food nutrients.

PREPARATION: Caribou, Sitka black-tail deer and reindeer can be boiled, roasted, grilled and dried

Caribou

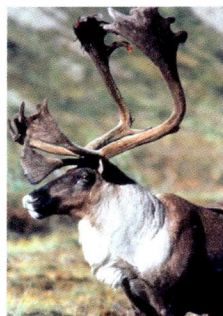

U.S. Fish & Wildlife Service

NATIVE NAMES: **Tuntuq** *(Yup'ik),* **Ghenuy** *(Dena'ina),* **Watsíx** *(Tlingit),* **Itx̂ayax̂** *(Unangam Tunuu),* **Tuttu** *(Iñupiaq)*

Caribou have been eaten in Alaska for thousands of years. They live in the tundra, muskeg and forests. Caribou are the only member of the deer family in which both sexes grow antlers. There are about one million caribou in Alaska. Herds numbering 350,000 animals can travel up to 900 miles during the summer from calving areas to wintering grounds. The liver, tongue, brain, blood and kidneys are delicacies that add valuable nutrients to the diet. Caribou has more protein and iron than the same amount of beef, and less of the unhealthy saturated fat.

Considered an important food of the Alaska Native people, almost all the parts of the caribou are eaten, including the tongue and bone marrow. Caribou is the only animal for which there were hunting songs, which came to the hunter as he awakened. People say that a caribou would "sing through" a person, either to let him know they were nearby or to reveal a taboo that had been broken.

40

CARIBOU NUTRITION INFORMATION

Caribou is an excellent source of protein & iron

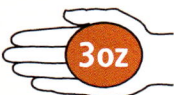

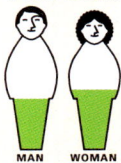

PROTEIN

MAN   WOMAN

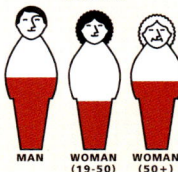

IRON

MAN   WOMAN (19-50)   WOMAN (50+)

HEART FRIENDLY
- Low in saturated fat
- Low in sodium

NUTRITION INFORMATION	
Per serving - 3 oz: cooked	
Calories	142
Protein	25 g
Carbohydrate	0 g
Fat	4 g
Calories from fat	25 %
Saturated fat	1 g
Dietary Fiber	0 g
Cholesterol	93 mg
Sodium	51 mg
Vitamin A	0
Vitamin C	3 mg
Iron	5 mg

Deer NATIVE NAMES: Tuntucuaq *(Yup'ik)*, Guwakaan *(Tlingit)*

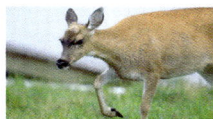

U.S. Fish & Wildlife Service

Sitka black-tailed deer can be found in two Alaska locations: the coastal forests of Southeast Alaska and on Kodiak Island. The Sitka black-tailed deer is smaller than the black-tailed deer, weighing between 80 to 100 pounds. The deer on Kodiak Island, however, are much larger and can weigh up to 200 pounds.

DEER NUTRITION INFORMATION

Deer is an excellent source of protein & iron

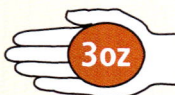

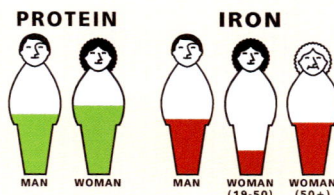

3oz

PROTEIN MAN WOMAN

IRON MAN WOMAN (19-50) WOMAN (50+)

HEART FRIENDLY
- Low in saturated fat
- Low in sodium

NUTRITION INFORMATION	
Per serving - 3 oz: cooked	
Calories	134
Protein	26 g
Carbohydrate	0 g
Fat	3 g
Calories from fat	20 %
Saturated fat	1 g
Dietary Fiber	0 g
Cholesterol	95 mg
Sodium	46 mg
Vitamin A	0
Vitamin C	0 mg
Iron	4 mg

41

Reindeer NATIVE NAMES: Qusngiq *(Yup'ik)*, Vejexshla *(Dena'ina)*, Itx̂aygix̂ *(Unangam Tunuu)*, Qunfiq *(Iñupiaq)*

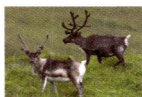

U.S. Fish & Wildlife Service

Domesticated reindeer were imported to Western Alaska from Siberia as a solution to the food shortage that resulted from unregulated whaling, which wiped out local populations of marine mammals. By federal regulation, only Alaska Native people are allowed to keep reindeer herds.

REINDEER NUTRITION INFORMATION

Reindeer is an excellent source of protein & iron

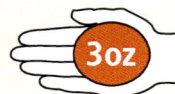

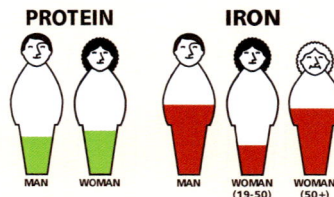

3oz

PROTEIN MAN WOMAN

IRON MAN WOMAN (19-50) WOMAN (50+)

HEART FRIENDLY
- Low in saturated fat
- Low in sodium

NUTRITION INFORMATION	
Per serving - 3 oz: raw	
Calories	107
Protein	19 g
Carbohydrate	0 g
Fat	3 g
Calories from fat	25 %
Saturated fat	1 g
Dietary Fiber	0 g
Cholesterol	13 mg
Sodium	NT*
Vitamin A	159 IU
Vitamin C	0 mg
Iron	5 mg

*Not Tested

Hare

Arctic Hare, Snowshoe Hare, Rabbit

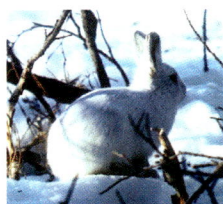

NATIVE NAMES: Maqaruaq *(Yup'ik)*, Ggeh *(Dena'ina)*, Gáx *(Tlingit)*, Uskaanax̂ *(Unangam Tunuu)*, Ukalliq -*Snowshoe (Iñupiaq)*

Hare is an important traditional food. It is found throughout the state and is hunted year-round. Hare rest in protected areas like thickets during the day. When threatened, they thump their hind feet on the ground as an alarm signal. The most commonly known hare in Alaska is the snowshoe.

PREPARATION: Hare or rabbit can be prepared much like poultry meat: roasted, broiled, grilled, fried, and stewed.

CAUTION: Care should be taken during the skinning and cleaning process as the disease tularemia, or "rabbit fever," is common in Alaskan hares; wear protective gloves and clean utensils with hot soapy water.

"They have deep, warm fur, but their skin is very fragile and easily torn . . . In former times they cut the hide spirally to make long strips, which they wove into garments or blankets. The overgrown, furry feet served as washcloths and dishrags, and children also made toy dogs of them."

– Prayers to the Raven, A Koyukon View of the Northern Forest

HARE NUTRITION INFORMATION

*nutrient data based on cooked wild rabbit

Hare is an excellent source of protein & iron

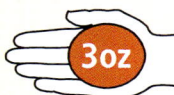

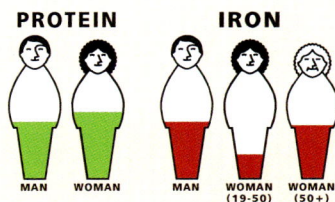

PROTEIN

IRON

MAN   WOMAN

MAN   WOMAN (19-50)   WOMAN (50+)

3oz

HEART FRIENDLY
- Low in saturated fat
- Low in sodium

NUTRITION INFORMATION	
Per serving - 3 oz: cooked	
Calories	147
Protein	28 g
Carbohydrate	0 g
Fat	3 g
Calories from fat	18 %
Saturated fat	1 g
Dietary Fiber	0 g
Cholesterol	105 mg
Sodium	38 mg
Vitamin A	0 IU
Vitamin C	0 mg
Iron	4 mg

Moose

NATIVE NAMES: Tuntuvak *(Yup'ik),* Dnigi *(Dena'ina),* Dzísk'w *(Tlingit),* Tuttuvak *(Iñupiaq)*

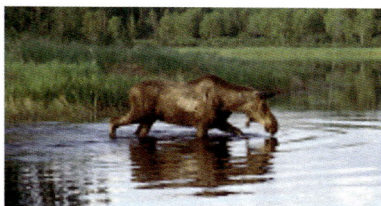

U.S. Fish & Wildlife Service

Moose is the most coveted and sought after meat among most Alaska Native populations. A moose may weigh between 800 to 1400 pounds. Moose heart, liver and nose are said to have no equal for tenderness and flavor.

PREPARATION: Moose meat can be eaten raw, frozen, boiled, baked, grilled, fried, or dried.

Alaska Native elders know how a moose was harvested by the taste and texture of its meat. If the moose is tough and strong tasting the hunter is often asked, "Why did you let it run?"

"When moose is out of season, we are still allowed to get one for memorial potlatches. Only men can cut up the meat for potlatches (moose/caribou). The moose parts saved for stew are the tongue, nose (shave hair off), and heart. To prepare, boil for 2-3 hours, add macaroni/rice, vegetables (potatoes/carrots), and canned tomatoes."
— *Audrey Armstrong, Huslia*

43

MOOSE NUTRITION INFORMATION

Moose is an excellent source of protein & iron

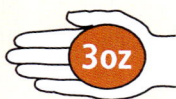

3oz

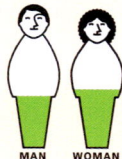

PROTEIN

MAN   WOMAN

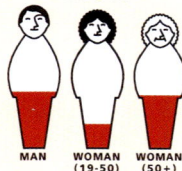

IRON

MAN   WOMAN (19-50)   WOMAN (50+)

HEART FRIENDLY
- Low in fat • Low in saturated fat
- Low in sodium

NUTRITION INFORMATION	
Per serving - 3 oz: cooked	
Calories	114
Protein	25 g
Carbohydrate	0 g
Fat	1 g
Calories from fat	8 %
Saturated fat	0 g
Dietary Fiber	0 g
Cholesterol	66 mg
Sodium	59 mg
Vitamin A	0
Vitamin C	4 mg
Iron	4 mg

Musk Ox

NATIVE NAMES: **Maankaaq** *(Yup'ik),* **Oomingmak** *(Iñupiaq)*

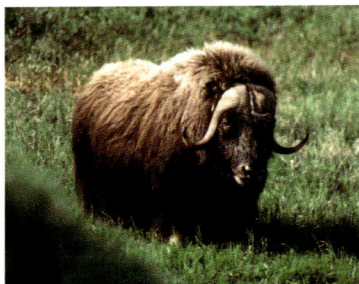
U.S. Fish & Wildlife Service

During prehistoric times, musk oxen wandered across the Bering Land Bridge to populate North America with the woolly mammoth, saber-toothed cat, and giant ground sloth. Musk oxen died off in Alaska in the late 1800s due to over-hunting. They were reintroduced in the 1930s from wild herds in Greenland and several thousand exist in the wild today. When threatened they protect their young by forming circles around them and facing outward.

PREPARATION: Musk Ox can be prepared much like moose: roasted, fried, grilled, boiled, and used in casserole dishes.

44

A layer of qiviut (pronounced KIV-EE-UTE) protects the animals from temperatures to -100° F. The wool is eight times warmer than sheep's wool by weight and is hand-knitted by Alaska Native people working in a cooperative arrangement into some of the most luxurious garments in the world. The wool can also be purchased in knitting stores.

MUSK OX NUTRITION INFORMATION*

*nutrient data based on bison

Musk ox is an excellent source of protein & a good source of iron

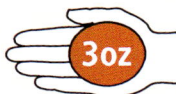

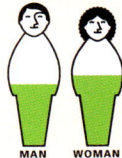
PROTEIN
MAN   WOMAN

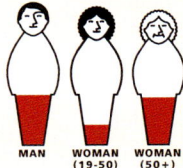
IRON
MAN   WOMAN (19-50)   WOMAN (50+)

HEART FRIENDLY
- Low in fat • Low in saturated fat
- Low in sodium

NUTRITION INFORMATION	
Per serving - 3 oz: cooked	
Calories	122
Protein	24 g
Carbohydrate	0 g
Fat	2 g
Calories from fat	15 %
Saturated fat	1 g
Dietary Fiber	0 g
Cholesterol	70 mg
Sodium	48 mg
Vitamin A	0
Vitamin C	0 mg
Iron	3 mg

Muskrat

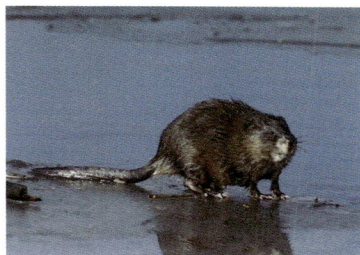

U.S. Fish & Wildlife Service

NATIVE NAMES: Kanaqlak *(Yup'ik)*, Tałtsuda *(Dena'ina)*, Tsín *(Tlingit)*, Kivgaluk *(Iñupiaq)*

Muskrat live throughout most of Alaska's mainland in flood plains and marshy areas. They mainly eat plants, so a muskrat's flesh is sweet and palatable. It is similar to rabbit, with darker meat.

PREPARATION: Muskrat can be roasted, fried, grilled, boiled, and used in casserole dishes. Muskrat is not good rare: it needs to be fully cooked.

"My mother would put fat and onions in the muskrat's stomach cavity and bake it until it was well done." — Elder

45

MUSKRAT NUTRITION INFORMATION

Muskrat is an excellent source of protein & iron

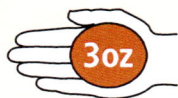

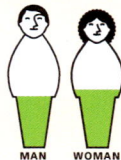

PROTEIN

MAN   WOMAN

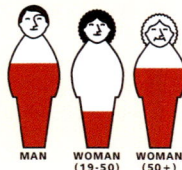

IRON

MAN   WOMAN (19-50)   WOMAN (50+)

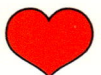

HEART FRIENDLY
● Low in sodium

NUTRITION INFORMATION	
Per serving - 3 oz: cooked	
Calories	199
Protein	26 g
Carbohydrate	0 g
Fat	10 g
Calories from fat	45 %
Saturated fat	NT*
Dietary Fiber	0 g
Cholesterol	103 mg
Sodium	81 mg
Vitamin A	0
Vitamin C	6 mg
Iron	6 mg

*Not Tested

Porcupine

NATIVE NAMES: Cukilek *(Yup'ik)*,
Qanchi *(Dena'ina)*, Xalak'ách' *(Tlingit)*,
Nuunix̂ *(Unangam Tunuu)*, Qirjaġluk *(Iñupiaq)*

The porcupine is found throughout Alaska,
except the Alaska Peninsula and Kodiak,
Nunivak, and St. Lawrence Islands. It
spends much of its time in spruce and
hemlock trees feeding on leaves, twigs and
bark. Since porcupines are slow moving,
they are easily caught. For this reason,
they are considered an emergency food.

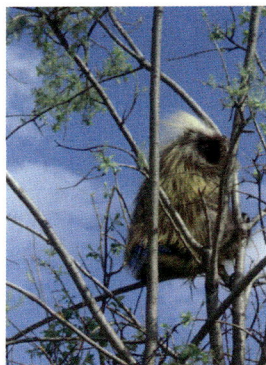

U.S. Fish & Wildlife Service

PREPARATION: Porcupine can be boiled, fried, roasted, and
used in stir fry dishes. Chew the meat slowly to avoid pieces of
quill. Porcupine meat is similar to pork.

*Athabascan Indians use porcupine quills to make jewelry and as
decoration on clothing. In former times, the "intestine" with fecal
pellets inside was dried and used for baby belts. It was believed that
it helped the baby have hard feces. This was important in the days
when moss was the only diaper.*

46

PORCUPINE NUTRITION INFORMATION*

*nutrient data based
on Raccoon

Porcupine is an
excellent source of
protein & iron

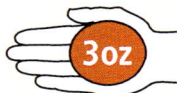

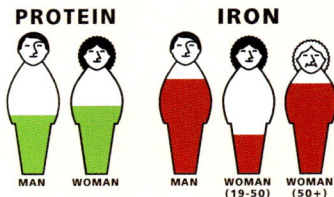

3oz

PROTEIN

MAN   WOMAN

IRON

MAN   WOMAN   WOMAN
       (19-50)   (50+)

HEART FRIENDLY
• Low in sodium

NUTRITION INFORMATION	
Per serving - 3 oz: cooked	
Calories	217
Protein	25 g
Carbohydrate	0 g
Fat	12 g
Calories from fat	50 %
Saturated fat	3 g
Dietary Fiber	0 g
Cholesterol	82 mg
Sodium	67 mg
Vitamin A	0
Vitamin C	0 mg
Iron	6 mg

Squirrel

NATIVE NAMES: Qanganaq *(Yup'ik)*, Deldida *(Dena'ina)*, Kals'áak *(Tlingit)*, Uulngiix̂ *(Unangam Tunuu)*, Siksrik *(Iñupiaq)*

There are two types of squirrels in Alaska: tree and ground. The ground squirrel primarily inhabits the mountains and tundra.

U.S. Fish & Wildlife Service

PREPARATION: Squirrel can be prepared by removing the small waxy scent glands inside the fore legs, and washing them completely to remove any loose hair. Squirrel can be broiled, baked, stewed, used in casseroles, roasted, and fried. The flesh of the squirrel has a medium red color, is tender, and has a wonderful taste.

"When I was a child, Native women trapped squirrels for the skin to make parkys for women and children. The skins were treasured as well as the meat. Women cleaned the squirrel, scraped the hide with their special tools and then dried them. It took a long time. Today, the squirrel skins are still used for parkys and are called 'parky squirrels.'"

– Nina Heavener, Clarks Point

47

SQUIRREL NUTRITION INFORMATION

Squirrel is an excellent source of protein & iron

3oz

PROTEIN MAN WOMAN

IRON MAN WOMAN (19-50) WOMAN (50+)

HEART FRIENDLY
- Low in saturated fat
- Low in sodium

NUTRITION INFORMATION	
Per serving - 3 oz: cooked	
Calories	147
Protein	26 g
Carbohydrate	0 g
Fat	4 g
Calories from fat	24 %
Saturated fat	1 g
Dietary Fiber	0 g
Cholesterol	103 mg
Sodium	101 mg
Vitamin A	0
Vitamin C	0 mg
Iron	6 mg

Bird Eggs
Sea Gull, Tern, Goose, Duck, Murre

NATIVE NAMES: **Kayanguq** *(Yup'ik)*,
K'eghaya *(Dena'ina)*, **K'wát'** *(Tlingit)*,
Mannik *(Iñupiaq)*

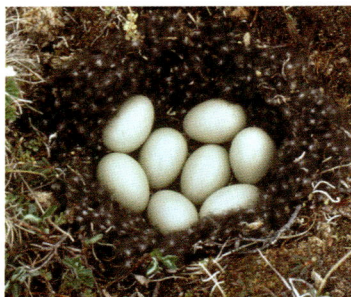

U.S. Fish & Wildlife Service

Seagull eggs are gray with spots
and are among the most popular
eggs to gather. Gulls lay more eggs when some
are taken from their nests. Goose, duck, and tern eggs are also
gathered, yet are smaller and harder to find. Eggs are usually
harvested from the last week in May until the second week in
June. Murre eggs are also popular in the Northwest regions of the
state and are harvested in July.

PREPARATION: Bird eggs can be prepared and used like
chicken eggs. For example, seagull and goose eggs are great in
cake mixes. Use one gull egg to replace one chicken egg. Boil eggs
in water for at least 20 minutes for hard-boiled eggs.

*To test if an egg is good to eat, Alaska Native people put it in water.
If it sinks, it is good to eat. If it floats, it is about to hatch and is
not good to eat.*

48

BIRD EGG NUTRITION INFORMATION

Bird eggs are a good
source Vitamin A,
protein & iron

(1egg)

IRON

MAN | WOMAN (19-50) | WOMAN (50+)

VITAMIN A

MAN | WOMAN

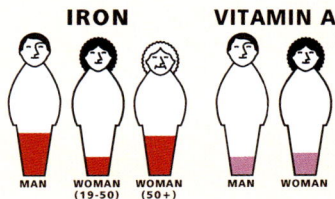

❤ **HEART FRIENDLY**
● Low in sodium

NUTRITION INFORMATION	
Per serving - 1 egg (duck)	
Calories	130
Protein	9 g
Carbohydrate	1 g
Fat	10 g
Calories from fat	69 %
Saturated fat	3 g
Dietary Fiber	0 g
Cholesterol	619 mg
Sodium	102 mg
Vitamin A	472 IU
Vitamin C	0 mg
Iron	3 mg

Black Brant

NATIVE NAMES:
Leqlernaq *(Yup'ik)*,
Chulyin Viy'a *(Dena'ina)*,
Kín *(Tlingit)*

U.S. Fish & Wildlife Service

Brants are the last of the geese and the fattest to arrive in Northwest Alaska each spring. They pass through Alaska when the lakes are still frozen but the rivers are flowing. Due to their soft meat and yellow fat, people enjoy eating them as soon as they arrive. The majority nest in the Yukon Delta. In addition, large concentrations of breeding brant are also found on the North Slope.

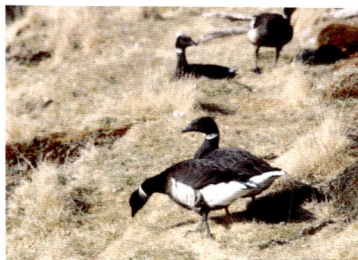

PREPARATION: Brant can be prepared much like chicken: roasted, baked, broiled, grilled, fried, or stewed. Brants also make great soups and casseroles.

The black brant seldom travels inland from the coast. In the Northwestern Interior it is named K'ideelgho nodaala, "goes the opposite way." It is no compliment when someone is described a being "just like K'ideelgho nodaala," implying a different or contrary approach to everything.

49

BLACK BRANT NUTRITION INFORMATION

Black Brant is an excellent source of protein and iron

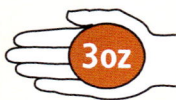

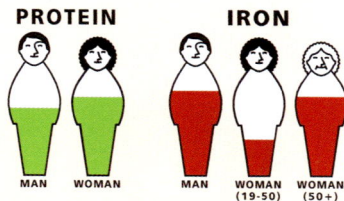

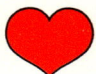

3oz

PROTEIN

MAN   WOMAN

IRON

MAN   WOMAN (19-50)   WOMAN (50+)

HEART FRIENDLY
• Very low in sodium

NUTRITION INFORMATION	
Per serving - 3 oz: raw	
Calories	151
Protein	28 g
Carbohydrate	1 g
Fat	4 g
Calories from fat	24 %
Saturated fat	2 g
Dietary Fiber	0 g
Cholesterol	88 mg
Sodium	30 mg
Vitamin A	0
Vitamin C	0 mg
Iron	6 mg

Canada Goose

NATIVE NAMES: Lagilugpiaq *(Yup'ik)*,
Nut'aq'i *(Dena'ina)*, T'aawák *(Tlingit)*,
Iqsraġutilik *(Iñupiaq)*

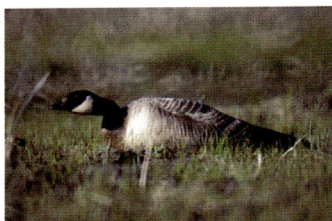

U.S. Fish & Wildlife Service

People enjoy seeing the geese return,
as it means the arrival of spring.
The sight of a flying "V" formation
and the sound of honking overhead is a sight
for tired winter eyes and ears. Geese are fast flappers and they are
generally eaten in the fall when they are fatter. A gander (male)
protecting the nest makes a formidable adversary. His wings are
capable of delivering a blow of surprising force, sufficient to scare
away a fox and similar predators. Canada geese mate for life.

PREPARATION: Goose can be prepared much like chicken:
roasted, baked, broiled, grilled, fried, or stewed. Goose also
makes great soups and casseroles. Traditionally they were boiled,
and eaten with seal oil or made into a soup.

50

*When geese call very noisily as they fly north in the spring, the
weather will turn warm; when they make little or no sound, it will
soon become cold.*

CANADA GOOSE NUTRITION INFORMATION

Canada goose is an
excellent source of
protein and a good
source of iron

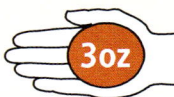

3oz

PROTEIN

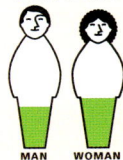

MAN   WOMAN

IRON

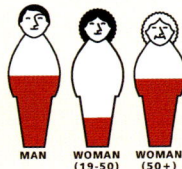

MAN   WOMAN   WOMAN
       (19-50)   (50+)

HEART FRIENDLY
● Low in sodium

NUTRITION INFORMATION	
Per serving - 3 oz	
Calories	139
Protein	19 g
Carbohydrate	0 g
Fat	6 g
Calories from fat	39 %
Saturated fat	2 g
Dietary Fiber	0 g
Cholesterol	71 mg
Sodium	74 mg
Vitamin A	NT*
Vitamin C	NT*
Iron	5 mg

*Not Tested

Crane

Sandhill Crane

NATIVE NAMES: Erinatuli *(Yup'ik)*,
Ndał *(Dena'ina)*, Dóol *(Tlingit)*, Tatirgak *(Iñupiaq)*

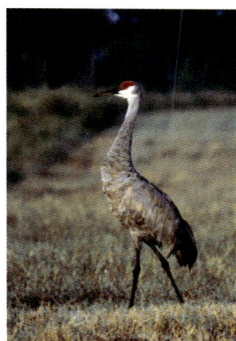

U.S. Fish & Wildlife Service

The sandhill crane breeds in the Yukon-Kuskokwim Delta, the Interior, and along coastal areas throughout Western and Northern Alaska. These birds, along with others from Siberia and Canada, are from the mid-continent population of cranes that winter in Texas, the Southwestern United States and Mexico. A smaller group, the Pacific Flyway, breeds in the Bristol Bay lowlands, on the Alaska Peninsula, and in the Cook Inlet and Susitna Valley region. A few nests have also been found in Southeast Alaska. Sandhill cranes are noted for their mating dance of deep bows followed by leaps, skips, and turns.

51

PREPARATION: Crane can be prepared much like chicken: roasted, baked, broiled, grilled, fried, or stewed. Crane also make great soups and casseroles.

The sandhill crane is Alaska's largest game bird. Residents of the Yukon-Kuskokwim Delta have affectionately nicknamed it the "Sunday Turkey."

– Alaska Department of Fish & Game

CRANE NUTRITION INFORMATION

Crane is an excellent source of protein & iron

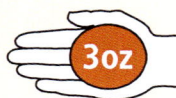

3oz

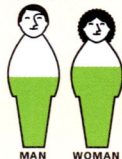

PROTEIN

MAN   WOMAN

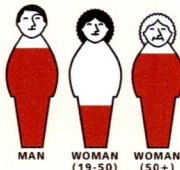

IRON

MAN   WOMAN (19-50)   WOMAN (50+)

HEART FRIENDLY
- Low in saturated fat
- Low in sodium

NUTRITION INFORMATION	
Per serving - 3 oz: raw	
Calories	135
Protein	29 g
Carbohydrate	0 g
Fat	2 g
Calories from fat	13 %
Saturated fat	1 g
Dietary Fiber	1 g
Cholesterol	106 mg
Sodium	47 mg
Vitamin A	0
Vitamin C	0 mg
Iron	6 mg

Duck

NATIVE NAMES: Atatek *(Yup'ik)*,
Dałishla *(Dena'ina)*, Gáaxw *(Tlingit)*,
Quagak *(Iñupiaq)*

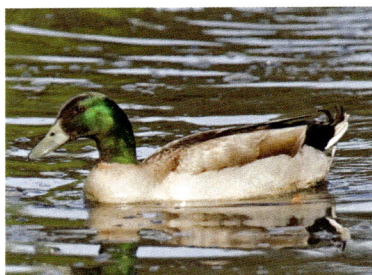

U.S. Fish & Wildlife Service

Ducks are mainly migratory
birds, present in the Northern
Regions of Alaska from May to
September. However, some duck
species, especially seaducks, remain all winter
in Southeast Alaska and other coastal, ice-free
areas. There are at least 39 different species of ducks in Alaska:
wigeon, mallard, shovelers, pintails, teal, scaup, eiders, harlequin
ducks, scoters, long-tailed ducks, goldeneye, and mergansers.
Duck meat is an excellent source of protein. Duck meat and eggs
provide important nutrients for health.

PREPARATION: Duck can be prepared much like chicken:
roasted, baked, broiled, grilled, fried, or stewed. Duck also makes
great soups and casseroles.

An elder suggests: "Boil the duck in soda and salt water for ten
minutes, wash it off and proceed with the stuffing and roasting
process."

*Green-winged teal ducks are found throughout Northwest Alaska
but were rarely hunted because they were so small. They are often
called "cup-a-soup" because of their size.*

DUCK NUTRITION INFORMATION

Duck is an excellent
source of protein &
iron

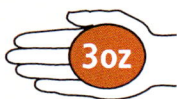

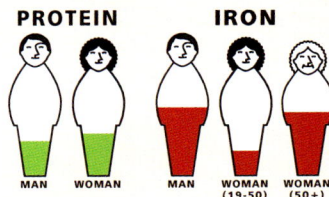

3oz

PROTEIN

MAN   WOMAN

IRON

MAN   WOMAN   WOMAN
      (19-50) (50+)

HEART FRIENDLY
• Low in sodium

NUTRITION INFORMATION	
Per serving - 3 oz: raw	
Calories	105
Protein	17 g
Carbohydrate	0
Fat	4 g
Calories from fat	34 %
Saturated fat	1 g
Dietary Fiber	0
Cholesterol	65 mg
Sodium	48 mg
Vitamin A	45 IU
Vitamin C	5 mg
Iron	4 mg

52

Ptarmigan

NATIVE NAMES: Qangqiiq *(Yup'ik)*, X'eis'awáa *(Tlingit)*

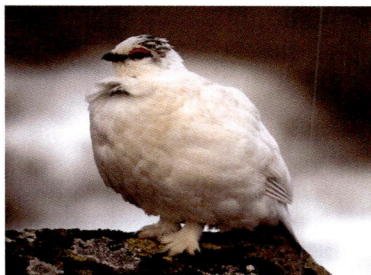

U.S. Fish & Wildlife Service

Unlike ducks and geese, ptarmigan live year-round in the north. They are known for coming and going. They seldom stay in one area for a long time. It is said when fox are around, ptarmigan move into the hills. Ptarmigan change color from brown to white during the winter months.

PREPARATION: Ptarmigan are considered very good to eat, and can be prepared much like chicken: roasted, baked, broiled, grilled, fried, or stewed.

Hunters report ptarmigan follow caribou, eating in places where caribou pawed through the snow to get to the berries and moss. Ptarmigan feathers are super absorbant and were traditionally used to clean things up, similar to how paper towels are used today.

53

PTARMIGAN NUTRITION INFORMATION

Ptarmigan is an excellent source of protein & iron and a good source of Vitamin A

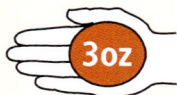

3oz

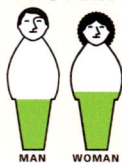

PROTEIN

MAN   WOMAN

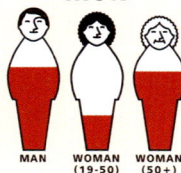

IRON

MAN   WOMAN (19-50)   WOMAN (50+)

HEART FRIENDLY
- Low in fat ● Low in saturated fat
- Low in cholesterol

NUTRITION INFORMATION	
Per serving - 3 oz: raw	
Calories	109
Protein	21 g
Carbohydrate	0 g
Fat	2 g
Calories from fat	16 %
Saturated fat	1 g
Dietary Fiber	NT*
Cholesterol	17 mg
Sodium	NT*
Vitamin A	357 IU
Vitamin C	NT*
Iron	5 mg

*Not Tested

"My dad took my son, Les, hunting and fishing. In the Eskimo way, when Les caught his first fish, everyone stopped to build a fire. The fish was cooked on a stick over the fire and the elders ate it. This meant that the elders now had a grandson who could care for them when they could no longer hunt and fish."

— Ruth Kalerak, Anchorage (originally from Solomon)

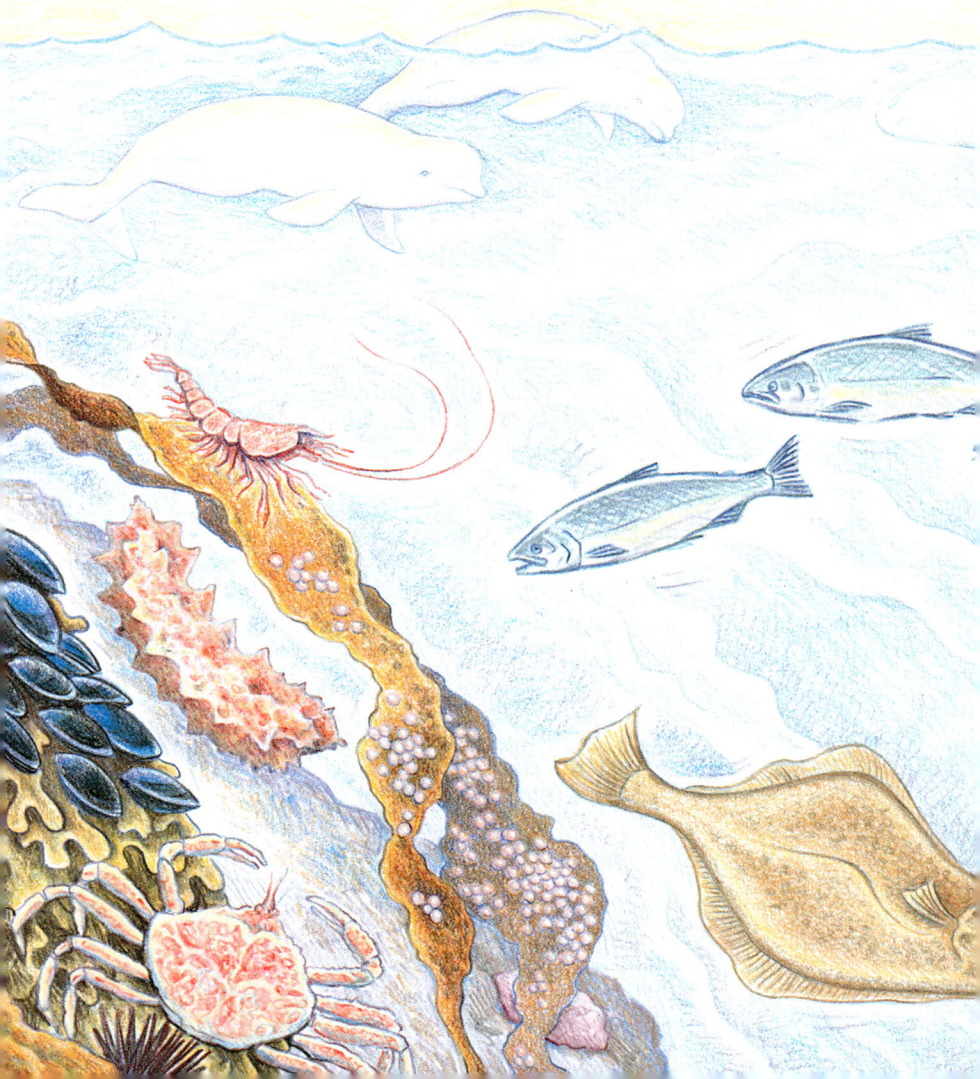

Food from the Sea

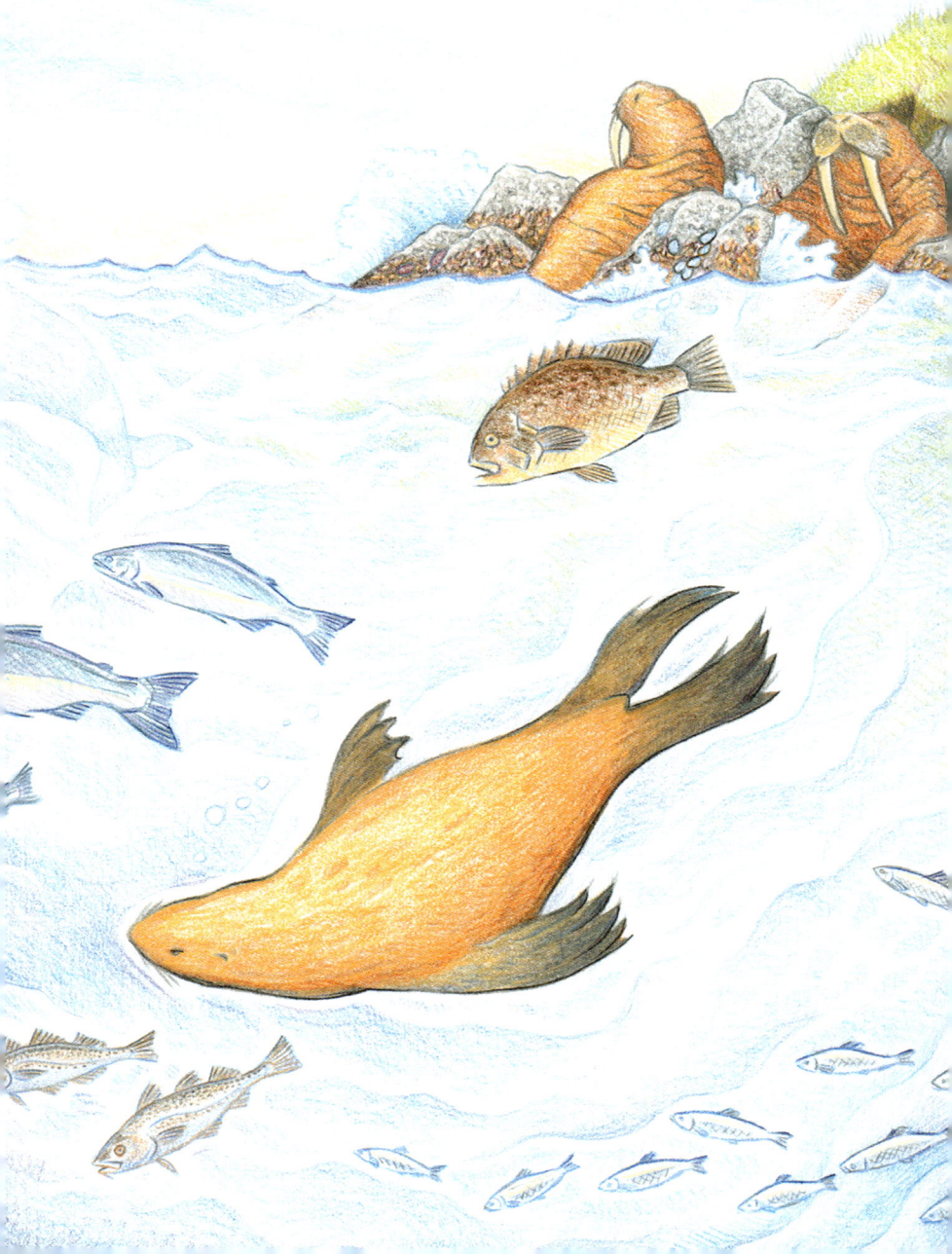

Abalone
(Northern & Pinto)

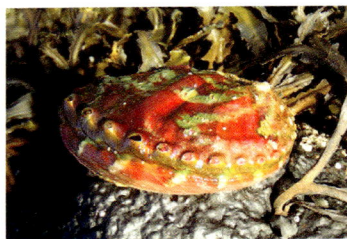

Marvin Scott

NATIVE NAMES:
Ivixuq or Uvixu - *snail (Iñupiaq)*,
Gúnxaa *(Tlingit)*

Abalone are part of the snail family. Although there are many types of abalone, Alaska has only one type, generally referred to as Northern or pinto (one of the smallest species found along the Pacific west coast). Abalone mature slowly and can grow to six inches in length. It is harvested along the coast in Southeast Alaska. Look for abalone during low tide along the bottom of rock ledges.

PREPARATION: Abalone can be eaten raw. It can be baked, boiled, fried, sautéed, or put in chowders and stews. Abalone can be preserved canned or frozen. Abalone meat toughens when overcooked. Its tenderness and flavor can be improved by storing in the refrigerator up to two days before it is prepared.

Abalone is a valued subsistence food in Haida and Tlingit communities in Southeast Alaska. Abalone shells have a brilliant pearl-like color and are used for totem poles, jewelry and traditional fish hooks.

56

ABALONE NUTRITION INFORMATION

Abalone is an excellent source of protein and a good source of iron

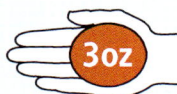

3oz

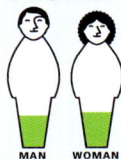

PROTEIN

MAN   WOMAN

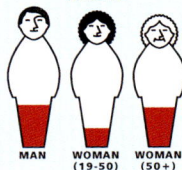

IRON

MAN   WOMAN (19-50)   WOMAN (50+)

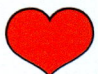

HEART FRIENDLY
- Low in fat
- Low in saturated fat

NUTRITION INFORMATION	
Per serving - 3 oz: raw	
Calories	89
Protein	15 g
Carbohydrate	5 g
Fat	1 g
Calories from fat	10 %
Saturated fat	0 g
Dietary Fiber	0 g
Cholesterol	72 mg
Sodium	256 mg
Vitamin A	6 IU
Vitamin C	2 mg
Iron	3 mg

Arctic Grayling

NATIVE NAMES:
Culugpauk *(Yup'ik)*,
Suluppaugaq *(Iñupiaq)*,
Ts'dat'ana *(Dena'ina)*,
Sulukpaugaq *(Iñupiaq)*

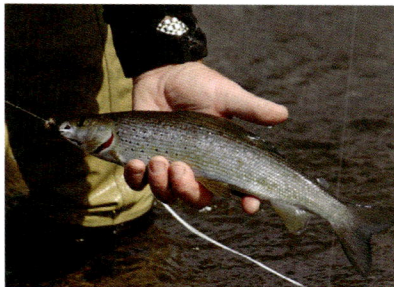

U.S. Fish & Wildlife Service

A relative of trout, Arctic grayling is a freshwater fish that weighs from one to three pounds. It is a migratory fish that can be found in lakes or medium-sized rivers such as the Chena and Gulkana, or in large glacial rivers like the Tanana, Susitna, and Yukon.

PREPARATION: Arctic grayling has an excellent white flaky flesh, usually eaten frozen (quaq), dried (paniqtuq) or cooked. The skin is good to eat, too.

Grayling have evolved to meet the needs of life in changing and harsh environments. They can be migratory or can complete their entire life in a short section of lake.

57

ARCTIC GRAYLING NUTRITION INFORMATION

Arctic grayling is an excellent source of protein

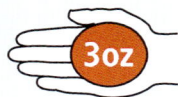

3oz

PROTEIN

MAN   WOMAN

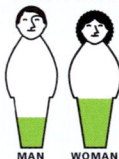

HEART FRIENDLY
- Low in fat
- Saturated fat free
- Low in sodium

NUTRITION INFORMATION	
Per serving - 3 oz	
Calories	79
Protein	17 g
Carbohydrate	0 g
Fat	1 g
Calories from fat	11 %
Saturated fat	0
Dietary Fiber	1 g
Cholesterol	49 mg
Sodium	69 mg
Vitamin A	<100 IU
Vitamin C	1 mg
Iron	1 mg

Black Cod
Sablefish

NATIVE NAMES:
Ceturrnaq *(Yup'ik),*
Ishkeen *(Tlingit)*

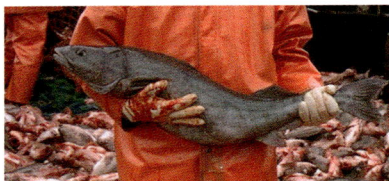

Alaska Fisheries Science Center,
NOAA Fisheries Service

Black cod is a saltwater whitefish. It is harvested from mid-March through mid-November. Black cod can grow up to ten pounds in weight and measure up to three feet in length. Alaska is considered the largest black cod source in the world.

PREPARATION: Black cod flesh is tender and has a rich, sweet flavor. Black cod can be baked, broiled, poached, sautéed, smoked, and steamed.

Black cod "tips" are considered a delicacy in Southeast Alaska. "The tip is the pectoral fin flesh, part of the bony collar just behind the head."

– The Alaska Heritage Seafood Cookbook

58

BLACK COD NUTRITION INFORMATION

*nutrient data based on Pacific Cod

Black cod is an excellent source of protein

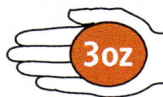

PROTEIN

MAN   WOMAN

3oz

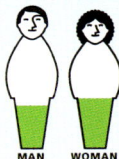

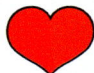

HEART FRIENDLY
- Low in fat • Saturated fat free
- Low in sodium

NUTRITION INFORMATION	
Per serving - 3 oz: cooked	
Calories	89
Protein	20 g
Carbohydrate	0
Fat	1 g
Calories from fat	10 %
Saturated fat	0
Dietary Fiber	0
Cholesterol	40 mg
Sodium	77 mg
Vitamin A	27 IU
Vitamin C	3 mg
Iron	0

Blackfish

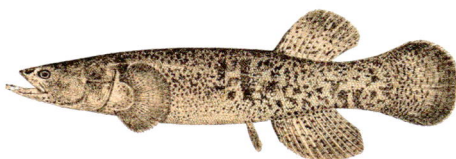

NATIVE NAMES:
Can'giiq *(Yup'ik)*,
Ijuuqieiq *(Iñupiaq)*, Huzhegh *(Dena'ina)*

Blackfish are only found in Alaska and Eastern Siberia. A bottom dwelling fish, it can grow up to eight inches in length. They typically live in the densely vegetated areas of lowland swamps, ponds, rivers, and lakes. Traditionally, blackfish has been eaten whole, including bones, which make them a good source of calcium.

PREPARATION: Blackfish are eaten frozen or cooked.

These tundra fish are most famous for being able to freeze as the water freezes and then return to life when the water thaws. "The best blackfish lakes are reported to be those with the most otter and mink sign."

– *Alaska Department of Fish & Game*

59

BLACKFISH NUTRITION INFORMATION

Blackfish is an excellent source of protein, iron and Vitamin A

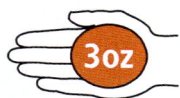

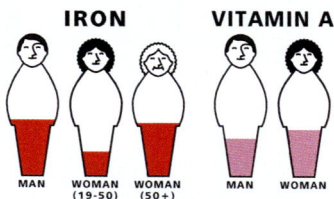

IRON

VITAMIN A

MAN WOMAN (19-50) WOMAN (50+) MAN WOMAN

HEART FRIENDLY
- Low in fat

NUTRITION INFORMATION	
Per serving - 3 oz: whole	
Calories	70
Protein	13 g
Carbohydrate	1 g
Fat	1 g
Calories from fat	19 %
Saturated fat	NT*
Dietary Fiber	NT*
Cholesterol	NT*
Sodium	NT*
Vitamin A	1022 IU
Vitamin C	NT*
Iron	4 mg

*Not Tested

Clams

NATIVE NAMES: **Aatevtaaq** *(Yup'ik),*
Tiq'adi *(Dena'ina),* **Gáal'** *(Tlingit),*
Imaniq *(Iñupiaq)*

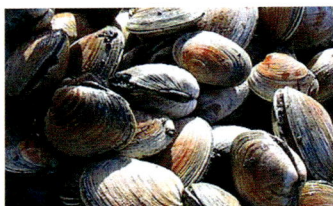

ANTHC

There are many species of clams
in Alaska. The more well known
varieties include razor (Arctic and Pacific),
butter, geoduck, and littleneck clams. They are gathered at low
tide during the summer and fall months. Look for a sandy beach
with holes or water squirting out and begin digging for clams.

**CAUTION: Alaska shellfish can become toxic due to
paralytic shellfish poisoning (PSP). Always check with
local fish and game officials before digging for clams.**

PREPARATION: Clams can be fried, steamed, or put in
chowder and dips. Clams can be canned, dried, frozen, or smoked.

*"My dad quit going clam digging. The whole family really enjoyed them.
But no one said anything to Daddy about why he quit until the beginning
of the third summer of not digging them. My sister asked him why he quit.
He said he hated cleaning them, and really missed digging them, but was
tired of cleaning them. My sister told him, 'Dad you dig them and I will
clean them.' So he did that for about five years (up until the summer before
he passed away). My sister said that was the best memory of our Dad
– just listening to his stories as they cleaned clams together. After they
completed the cleaning they would sit down for a bowl of clam chowder."*

– Selma Oskolkoff Simon, Anchorage

60

CLAMS NUTRITION INFORMATION

Clams are an excellent
source of protein
& iron

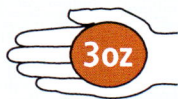

PROTEIN

IRON

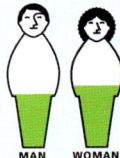

MAN   WOMAN

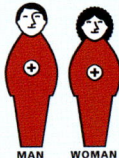

MAN   WOMAN

HEART FRIENDLY
- Low in fat • Saturated fat free
- Low in sodium

NUTRITION INFORMATION	
Per serving - 3 oz: cooked	
Calories	126
Protein	22 g
Carbohydrate	4 g
Fat	2 g
Calories from fat	12 %
Saturated fat	0 g
Dietary Fiber	NT*
Cholesterol	57 mg
Sodium	95 mg
Vitamin A	145 IU
Vitamin C	1 mg
Iron	24 mg
*Not Tested	

Cockles
Heart Clam

NATIVE NAMES: Tavtaaq *(Yup'ik)*

Cockles are a variety of clam found along the Bering Sea coast. Look for cockles just below the sand's surface. The more well known varieties in Alaska include the Basket, Northern,

Douglas Island Pink & Chum, Inc.

Nuttalls, Greenland, and Iceland cockles. Cockles are also known as the "heart clam" because of its shape when viewed from the side.

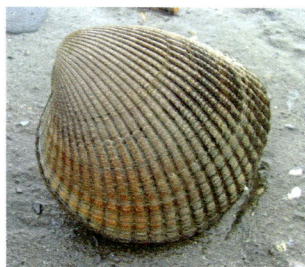

CAUTION: Alaska shellfish can become toxic due to paralytic shellfish poisoning (PSP). Always check with local fish and game officials before digging for cockles.

PREPARATION: Cockles can be eaten raw or preserved in salt and vinegar. They perish easily, so they should be cooked if not eaten right away. Cockles can be prepared much like clams: boiled, fried, roasted, steamed, or put in dips. Cockles can also be canned or frozen.

61

"Cockles, along with clams and chitons, were important backup foods for the Tlingit and Haida during 'starving times'--those lean winter months when fresh foods were unavailable and supplies of dried fish and dried clams had been exhausted."

– The Alaska Heritage Seafood Cookbook

COCKLES NUTRITION INFORMATION

Cockles are an excellent source of protein & iron

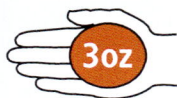

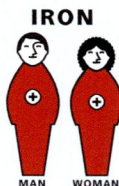

IRON

3oz

MAN   WOMAN

HEART FRIENDLY
- Low in fat

NUTRITION INFORMATION	
Per serving - 3 oz	
Calories	67
Protein	11 g
Carbohydrate	4 g
Fat	1 g
Calories from fat	8 %
Saturated fat	NT*
Dietary Fiber	NT*
Cholesterol	NT*
Sodium	NT*
Vitamin A	NT*
Vitamin C	NT*
Iron	14 mg

*Not Tested

Cod

NATIVE NAMES: **Atgiaq** *(Yup'ik),*
Hey Tsagela *(Dena'ina),*
Uugaq *- Tomcod (Iñupiaq),*
Atxida *(Unangam Tunuu),*
Chudéi *- Tomcod (Tlingit)*

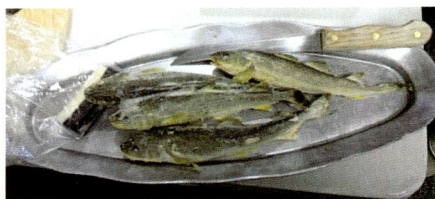

ANTHC

Several types of cod are eaten in Alaska, including tomcod and mudsharks. Cod is harvested in the Bering Sea and Gulf of Alaska, and is typically frozen as soon as it is caught.

PREPARATION: Cod can be baked, broiled, poached, fried, or steamed.

"Traditionally we took the insides out of the mudsharks and cut the whole fish up, including the skin, fins and head, and boiled it along with the eggs and liver. We grew up eating those fish and we learned to love that distinct taste. Sometimes, we yearn for it yet."

— Anore Jones

62

COD NUTRITION INFORMATION

Cod is an excellent source of protein

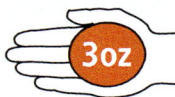

3oz

PROTEIN

MAN   WOMAN

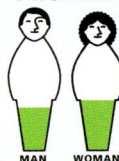

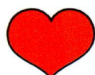

HEART FRIENDLY
- Low in fat • Saturated fat free
- Low in sodium

NUTRITION INFORMATION	
Per serving - 3 oz: cooked	
Calories	89
Protein	20 g
Carbohydrate	0
Fat	1 g
Calories from fat	10 %
Saturated fat	0
Dietary Fiber	0
Cholesterol	40 mg
Sodium	77 mg
Vitamin A	27 IU
Vitamin C	3 mg
Iron	0

Crab

NATIVE NAMES: Ivalriiyak *(Yup'ik),*
Ch'naɬ'in *(Dena'ina),*
S'áaw - *Dungeness (Tlingit),*
Puyyugiaq *(Iñupiaq)*

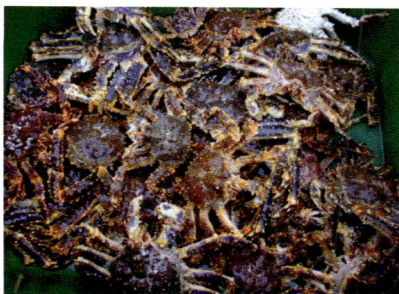

Carin Bailey

There are many species of
crab in Alaska. The more
well known varieties include
dungeness (dungies), king
(golden, blue, and red), and snow (also known
as tanner crab). King crabs are the largest, and their size can span
up to six feet in length. Snow crabs are one of the smaller crabs.
The legs of the crab have the most meat, with the body having
a small amount. Crabs are harvested in pots in the Bristol Bay,
Pribilof Islands, Norton Sound areas, and Southeast Alaska.

PREPARATION: Crab can be steamed, baked, simmered, or
boiled, and used in casseroles, salads, appetizers and sauces.

*The hazardous working conditions and weather make Alaska's crab
fisheries one of the most dangerous jobs in America.*

63

CRAB NUTRITION INFORMATION

*nutrient data based on King Crab

Crab is an excellent source of protein

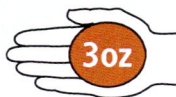

3 oz

PROTEIN

MAN   WOMAN

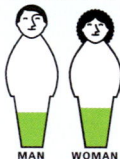

HEART FRIENDLY
- Low in fat
- Saturated fat free

NUTRITION INFORMATION	
Per serving - 3 oz: cooked	
Calories	82
Protein	16 g
Carbohydrate	0
Fat	1 g
Calories from fat	11 %
Saturated fat	0
Dietary Fiber	0
Cholesterol	45 mg
Sodium	911 mg
Vitamin A	25 IU
Vitamin C	7 mg
Iron	1 mg

Eulachon
Ooligan, Hooligan, Smelt

NATIVE NAMES:
Cemerliq or **Cimigliq** *(Yup'ik)*,
Dilhi *(Dena'ina)*,
Afmaksraq - *Smelt (Iñupiaq)*

Eulachon are slender, silver, shallow-water fish and can be found in both fresh and salt water across most of Alaska's coastline. Several types of smelt are eaten in Alaska, and are caught in dip nets, seines, and gill nets.

PREPARATION: Smelt can be boiled, baked, grilled, smoked, dried, and salted.

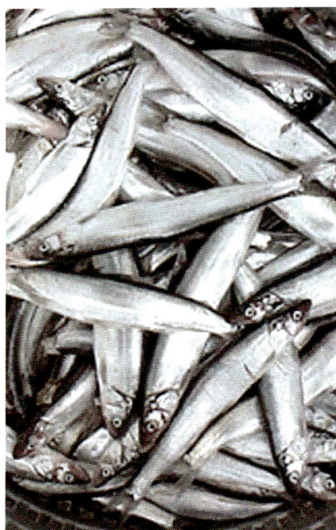

Alaska Fisheries Science Center, NOAA Fisheries Service

64

The extracted fat from hooligan, known as hooligan grease, is widely used as a condiment as well as a Native medicine, used traditionally for rashes. The Tsimshian Indians refer to eulachon ooligan as "savior fish," since it was the first fresh fish to return to Alaska in the spring. The people of Southeast Alaska refer to it as candle fish due to its high oil content, enough to make a "candle."

EULACHON NUTRITION INFORMATION

Eulachon is an excellent source of protein

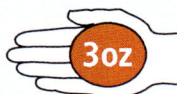

3oz

PROTEIN

MAN   WOMAN

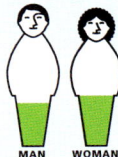

HEART FRIENDLY
- Saturated fat free
- Low in sodium

NUTRITION INFORMATION	
Per serving - 3 oz: cooked	
Calories	105
Protein	19 g
Carbohydrate	0
Fat	3 g
Calories from fat	23 %
Saturated fat	0
Dietary Fiber	0
Cholesterol	76 mg
Sodium	65 mg
Vitamin A	49 IU
Vitamin C	0
Iron	1 mg

Flounder

NATIVE NAMES:
Cagiq *(Yup'ik)*,
Hnighelq'ayi *(Dena'ina)*,
Dzánti *(Tlingit)*,
Nataaġnaq *(Iñupiaq)*

Flounder is a bottom dwelling flat fish similar to the halibut. Flounder can grow up to 10 pounds in weight. Species include "lemon sole," arrowtooth (turbot), blackback, dover and rock sole. Alaska is considered the largest flounder source in the world, with the largest numbers harvested in the Gulf of Alaska.

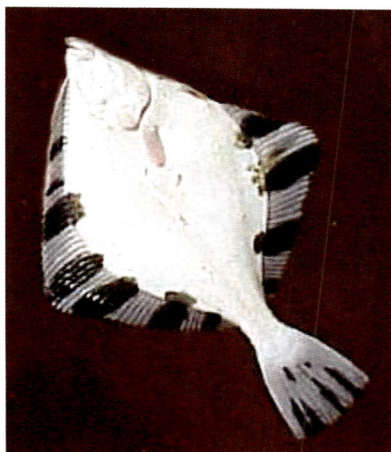

Alaska Fisheries Science Center, NOAA Fisheries Service

PREPARATION: Flounder can be baked, broiled, poached, fried, steamed, and dried or frozen.

65

FLOUNDER NUTRITION INFORMATION

Flounder is an excellent source of protein

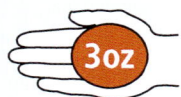

3 oz

PROTEIN

MAN   WOMAN

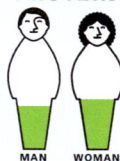

HEART FRIENDLY
- Low in fat • Saturated fat free
- Low in sodium

NUTRITION INFORMATION	
Per serving - 3 oz: cooked	
Calories	100
Protein	21 g
Carbohydrate	0 g
Fat	1 g
Calories from fat	9 %
Saturated fat	0 g
Dietary Fiber	0 g
Cholesterol	58 mg
Sodium	89 mg
Vitamin A	37 IU
Vitamin C	0
Iron	0s

Gumboots
Leathery Chiton, Bidarkis

NATIVE NAMES: Shaaw *(Tlingit)*

There are seven species of gumboots in Alaska, and the two more well known varieties include the black and giant chitons. An oval shaped mollusk with a black top, gumboots can measure up to ten inches in length. Gumboots attach themselves to the bottom of rocks and can be found in middle to lower tidal areas along the Aleutian Islands, Prince William Sound area, and Southeast Alaska.

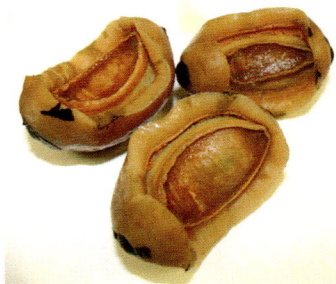

Alma Callis

PREPARATION: Gumboot meat has a sweet taste. Remove the inside brown strip of the gumboot and discard. The remaining meat can be eaten raw, boiled, dried, fried, pickled, roasted, or steamed. Gumboots taste good dipped in butter, added to chowders, or made into fish patties.

Gumboots are a prized food to the Tlingit, Haida, and Tsimshian.

Gumboot determination recognizes the gumboots "stick-to-it tenacity." Characterizing "gumboot determination" captures not only the purpose and strength of this small creature, but describes how the Alaska Native people of Southeast Alaska survived and overcame epidemics. – Gumboot Determination: The Story of the SouthEast Alaska Regional Health Consortium

GUMBOOT NUTRITION INFORMATION

Gumboot is an excellent source of protein, iron & Vitamin A

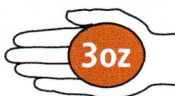

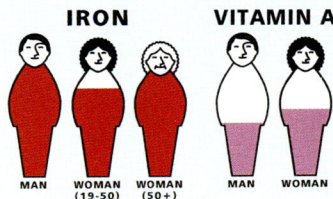

3oz

IRON

MAN | WOMAN (19-50) | WOMAN (50+)

VITAMIN A

MAN | WOMAN

HEART FRIENDLY
• Low in fat

NUTRITION INFORMATION	
Per serving - 3 oz	
Calories	71
Protein	15 g
Carbohydrate	0
Fat	1 g
Calories from fat	13 %
Saturated fat	NT*
Dietary Fiber	NT*
Cholesterol	NT*
Sodium	NT*
Vitamin A	1402 IU
Vitamin C	
Iron	14 mg

*Not Tested

Halibut

NATIVE NAMES: **Caqig** *(Yup'ik)*,
Taghelq'ayi *(Dena'ina)*, **Cháatl** *(Tlingit)*

Halibut is the largest of the flat fish and grows to over 600 pounds. The species tends to inhabit deep ocean waters and must be brought carefully to the surface to be kept alive. Alaska Natives once fished for halibut with wooden hooks suspended below floats made from seal stomachs. Their fishing line was made from cedar bark, spruce roots, kelp and other natural materials.

PREPARATION: Halibut can be baked, broiled, poached, fried, or steamed. The meat from the bottom of the halibut is used in soups and chowders, and the top side for steaks.

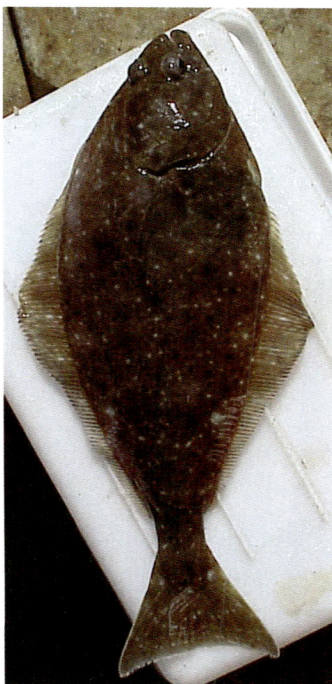

67

Alaska Fisheries Science Center, NOAA Fisheries Service

Salmon, Arctic char, halibut and pike skins were commonly used to create waterproof clothing and other household items such as storage containers. This reinforces traditional Alaska Native values that everything provided by nature must be put to good use.

HALIBUT NUTRITION INFORMATION

Halibut is an excellent source of protein

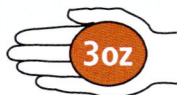

3oz

PROTEIN

MAN   WOMAN

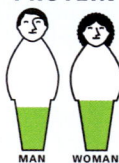

HEART FRIENDLY
- Low in fat • Saturated fat free
- Low in sodium

NUTRITION INFORMATION	
Per serving - 3 oz: cooked with skin	
Calories	96
Protein	19 g
Carbohydrate	0
Fat	2 g
Calories from fat	19 %
Saturated fat	0
Dietary Fiber	0
Cholesterol	64 mg
Sodium	73 mg
Vitamin A	136 IU
Vitamin C	NT*
Iron	0
*Not Tested	

Herring

NATIVE NAMES:
Iqalluarpak *(Yup'ik)*,
Kuts'enelkuha *(Dena'ina)*,
Yaaw *(Tlingit)*,
Uqsruqtuuq *(Iñupiaq)*

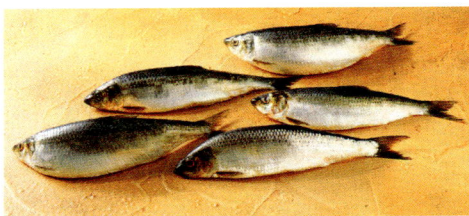

Alaska Seafood Marketing Institute

Herring move offshore to feed in the summer and become extremely fat in the fall. They move in-shore over winter where fresh water meets salt water. Herring are often harvested with the use of a gill net, but can be caught by jigging with a small, barbless, single hook or other sports gear.

PREPARATION: The most common way herring is eaten is baked or fried, preferably the day it is caught. Herring can also be dried, pickled, salted, or frozen.

"Last time someone seined herring, the net was so full and heavy that they had to turn one end loose and let them all go. It was too heavy to pull in."

– Kivalina resident

"Traditional dried herring remains a major staple of the diet in Bering Sea villages near Nelson Island where salmon are not readily available."

– Alaska Department of Fish and Game

68

HERRING NUTRITION INFORMATION

Herring is an excellent source of protein

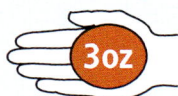

3oz

PROTEIN

MAN   WOMAN

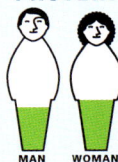

HEART FRIENDLY
● Low in sodium

NUTRITION INFORMATION	
Per serving - 3 oz: cooked	
Calories	212
Protein	18 g
Carbohydrate	0
Fat	15 g
Calories from fat	64 %
Saturated fat	4 g
Dietary Fiber	0
Cholesterol	84 mg
Sodium	81 mg
Vitamin A	99 IU
Vitamin C	0
Iron	1 mg

Herring Eggs

NATIVE NAMES: **Elquaq** *(Yup'ik)*,
Kuts'enelkuha Q'in *(Dena'ina)*,
Gáax'w *(Tlingit)*

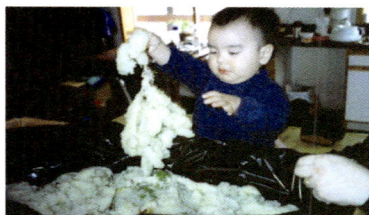

Mike and Edna Jackson

Herring eggs are considered an Alaska Native delicacy and sometimes called "Tlingit caviar." They are harvested either on ribbon kelp or hemlock branches submerged in an area where herring are known to spawn. The herring may be herded into the area and penned with nets to force them to spawn on the kelp or hemlock. Once enough eggs are deposited, the herring are released from the pen to spawn again for future harvests.

PREPARATION: Herring eggs are eaten raw or poached, with butter, seal oil, eulachon oil, or soy sauce. Herring eggs can also be dried.

Herring eggs will keep in the freezer for up to a year. It is best to thaw the eggs in a bowl of salt water, to help them defrost faster and dislodge sand from the eggs. Some Tlingit are connoisseurs of herring eggs, and know certain regions by their flavor or texture. Good harvest grounds are often jealously guarded secrets. Bristol Bay residents believe "3rd pass" (the third spawning) of herring eggs is the best.

69

HERRING EGG NUTRITION INFORMATION

Herring eggs are a good source of protein

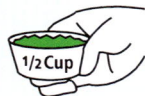

PROTEIN

MAN   WOMAN

1/2 Cup

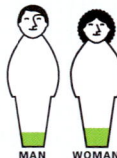

HEART FRIENDLY
- Low in fat • Saturated fat free
- Low in sodium

NUTRITION INFORMATION	
Per serving - 1/2 cup: raw	
Calories	63
Protein	8 g
Carbohydrate	4 g
Fat	2 g
Calories from fat	29 %
Saturated fat	0
Dietary Fiber	NT*
Cholesterol	34 mg
Sodium	52 mg
Vitamin A	48 IU
Vitamin C	1 mg
Iron	2 mg

*Not Tested

Hooligan Grease

NATIVE NAMES:
Saak eexÍ *(Tlingit)*

Hooligan (eulachon, ooligan, smelts) is an oily fish, and the oil rendered from it is primarily used as a dip for other foods. It is also used to preserve berries, roots, herbs, and salmon eggs. The oil has a clear color when prepared.

PREPARATION: Hooligan grease preparation varies. It can be frozen or kept in a jar in a cool place. Hooligan grease is used as a dip for dried fish, dried herring, or black seaweed. It can also be added to boiled fish and meat dishes.

Traditionally, hooligan grease was used as an indicator for weather changes, and social or personal events. An increased milky appearance in the grease predicted stormy weather for fishermen. Any fish parts remaining after the oil was rendered was often discarded into the river, and it was thought it would contribute nutrients [back to the river].

— www.nativeknowledge.org

70

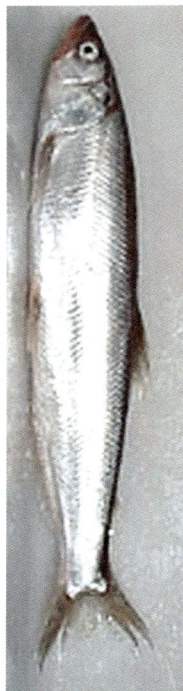

Alaska Fisheries Science Center, NOAA Fisheries Service

HOOLIGAN GREASE NUTRITION INFORMATION

*nutrient data based on euchalon grease

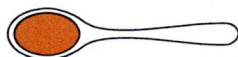

NUTRITION INFORMATION	
Per serving - 1 tablespoon	
Calories	135
Protein	0
Carbohydrate	0
Fat	15 g
Calories from fat	100 %
Saturated fat	4 g
Dietary Fiber	0
Cholesterol	0
Sodium	0
Vitamin A	848 IU
Vitamin C	0
Iron	0

Lingcod

NATIVE NAMES: X'áax'w *(Tlingit)*

Lingcod is different from cod and is classified as a greenling, a spiny-finned fish. Lingcod are slender and have a large head and mouth with very sharp teeth. They are a bottom dwelling fish and can be found near the rocky reefs of the Alaska Peninsula, Aleutian Islands, Southeast Alaska, and the outer Kenai Peninsula, Kodiak, and Prince William Sound areas. They can grow up to 80 pounds in weight and measure up to 60 inches in length.

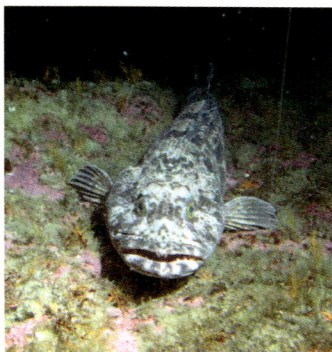

Alaska Department of Fish and Game Groundfish Project

PREPARATION: Lingcod flesh is a bluish color when raw, and turns white when cooked. Lingcod can be baked, broiled, fried, sautéed, and used in stews.

Lingcod liver and cheeks are considered a delicacy.

71

LINGCOD NUTRITION INFORMATION

Lingcod is an excellent source of protein

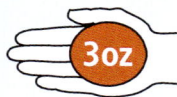

3oz

PROTEIN

MAN   WOMAN

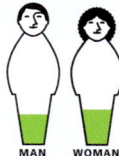

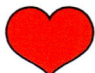

HEART FRIENDLY
- Low in fat • Saturated fat free
- Low in sodium

NUTRITION INFORMATION	
Per serving - 3 oz	
Calories	71
Protein	15 g
Carbohydrate	0
Fat	1 g
Calories from fat	8 %
Saturated fat	NT*
Dietary Fiber	NT*
Cholesterol	NT*
Sodium	50 mg
Vitamin A	196 IU
Vitamin C	NT*
Iron	NT*

*Not Tested

Octopus

NATIVE NAMES: **Amikuk** *(Yup'ik),* **Amaguk** *(Dena'ina)*

Octopus are a relative of clams, snails, and oysters. There are more than 30 different species of octopus that can weigh up to 100 pounds. The giant Pacific octopus is the largest and can grow to 30 feet in length. Octopus can be found along seaside cliffs at low tide or by overturning stones on outer flats during low tides.

CAUTION: be sure to handle the octopus carefully to avoid being bitten.

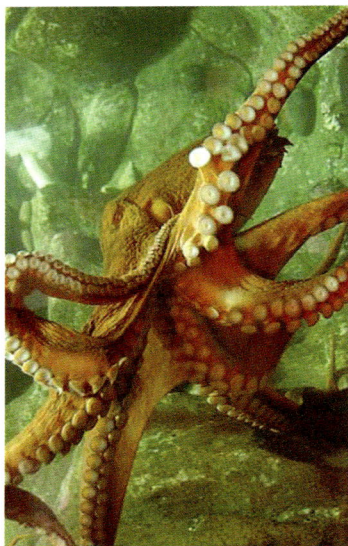

Alaska SeaLife Center

PREPARATION: Remove contents from inside the octopus's head as this is all waste. Clean tentacles of slime. This can be done by washing very thoroughly with slightly salted water. Too much salt will toughen the meat.

72

"Alaska's Aleut and Tlingit peoples relied on foods like octopus when game, fish, or large marine mammals were scarce. Octopus commonly wound up simmering in traditional chowders."

– Alaska Heritage Seafood Cookbook

OCTOPUS NUTRITION INFORMATION

Octopus is an excellent source of protein & iron

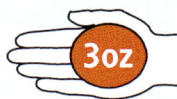

3oz

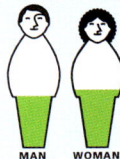

PROTEIN

MAN   WOMAN

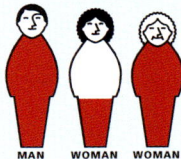

IRON

MAN   WOMAN (19-50)   WOMAN (50+)

HEART FRIENDLY
- Low in fat
- Saturated fat free

NUTRITION INFORMATION	
Per serving - 3 oz: cooked	
Calories	139
Protein	25 g
Carbohydrate	4 g
Fat	2 g
Calories from fat	13 %
Saturated fat	0
Dietary Fiber	0
Cholesterol	82 mg
Sodium	391 mg
Vitamin A	255 IU
Vitamin C	7 mg
Iron	8 mg

Pike

NATIVE NAMES:
Cuukvak *(Yup'ik)*,
Ghelguts'i *(Dena'ina)*,
Siulik *(Iñupiaq)*

Northern pike are a large fish ranging in weight from five to 50 pounds. They live in shallow lakes, streams, sloughs, and rivers. Pike is not a prized food, but it is eaten for variety or when other fish are not available.

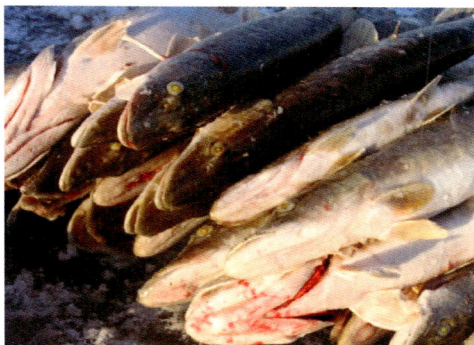

Donald Zanoff

PREPARATION: Northern pike are eaten dried, frozen, boiled, roasted, or fried and can be added to agutak. The skin of the pike has large scales and a heavy mucous. Some bake the fish in a heavy brown paper bag to allow the scales and skin to cling to the paper while cooking, leaving the tender meat intact. The pike's stomach, intestines, air bladder liner, and head are edible.

73

In the Distant Time, the pike ate a little baby that had just been fed from his mother's breast. The baby became the pike's liver and this is why a white fluid comes from pike liver when it is cooking.

PIKE NUTRITION INFORMATION

Pike is an excellent source of protein

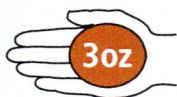

PROTEIN

3oz

MAN   WOMAN

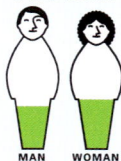

HEART FRIENDLY
- Low in fat • Saturated fat free
- Low in sodium

NUTRITION INFORMATION	
Per serving - 3 oz: cooked	
Calories	96
Protein	21 g
Carbohydrate	0 g
Fat	1 g
Calories from fat	9 %
Saturated fat	0
Dietary Fiber	0
Cholesterol	42 mg
Sodium	42 mg
Vitamin A	69 IU
Vitamin C	3.2 mg
Iron	1 mg

Chum Salmon

Dog fish

NATIVE NAMES: Iqaalluk *(Yup'ik),*
Seyi *(Dena'ina),* Téel' *(Tlingit),*
Qalugruaq *(Iñupiaq)*

Chum salmon have the widest
distribution of all the Pacific salmon.
Chum salmon are large fish which
provide many pounds of food (fresh,
dried and frozen). Bright silver
chums, fresh from the ocean, have the

Alaska Seafood Marketing Institute

most fat, the best color and the firmest flesh. As they move up
the river they use up some fat, making them easier to dry.

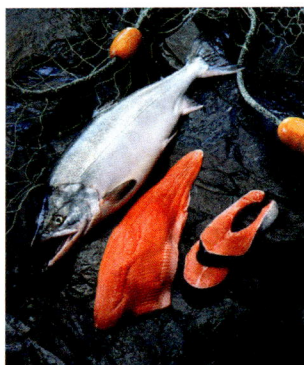

PREPARATION: Chum salmon can be dried, boiled half
dried, half dried and stored in seal oil, smoked, salted or pickled.
The eggs are also eaten in soup, raw and lightly fermented as
caviar, stored in oil or dried.

74

*"When salmon are half dead, those old, spawning salmon, their
skins are tough. We make water boots from this tough salmon skin."*
– Mamie Beaver in "Fish That We Eat"

CHUM SALMON
NUTRITION INFORMATION

Chum salmon is an excellent source of
protein

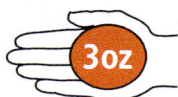

3oz

PROTEIN

MAN   WOMAN

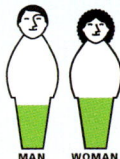

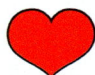

HEART FRIENDLY
- Low in saturated fat
- Low in sodium

NUTRITION INFORMATION	
Per serving - 3 oz: cooked	
Calories	131
Protein	22 g
Carbohydrate	0 g
Fat	4 g
Calories from fat	27 %
Saturated fat	1 g
Dietary Fiber	0
Cholesterol	81 mg
Sodium	54 mg
Vitamin A	97 IU
Vitamin C	0
Iron	1 mg

King Salmon

Chinook

NATIVE NAMES:
Taryakvak *(Yup'ik)*,
Łiq'a Ka'a *(Dena'ina)*,
T'á *(Tlingit)*,
Iqalugruaq *(Iñupiaq)*

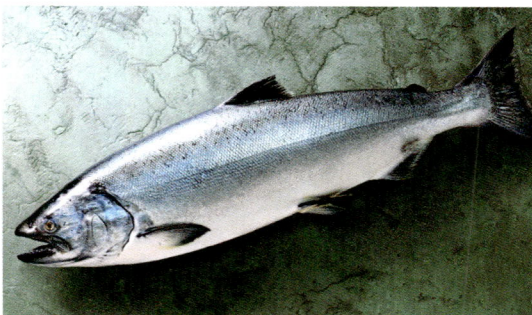
Alaska Seafood Marketing Institute

The largest of all salmon, kings weigh up to 40 pounds. They are prized for their red flesh, rich flavor, high-oil content, and firm texture. Subsistence fishermen in the Yukon and Kuskokwim Rivers catch an average of 60,000 kings per year.

PREPARATION: King salmon can be baked, broiled, grilled, fried, steamed, or poached. It can be used in casseroles and various other dishes. They may also be smoked, brined and dried in strips.

Salmon are more powerful than any other fish. Children may be sheltered from the danger of "bad spirits" by wearing dried salmon tails around their neck or carrying them in their pockets.

KING SALMON NUTRITION INFORMATION

King salmon is an excellent source of protein

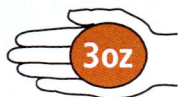

3oz

PROTEIN

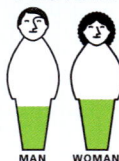

MAN   WOMAN

NUTRITION INFORMATION	
Per serving - 3 oz: kippered	
Calories	178
Protein	20 g
Carbohydrate	0
Fat	11 g
Calories from fat	56 %
Saturated fat	2 g
Dietary Fiber	0
Cholesterol	57 mg
Sodium	740 mg
Vitamin A	35 IU
Vitamin C	0
Iron	0

Pink Salmon
Humpback

NATIVE NAMES:
Amaqaayak *(Yup'ik),*
Łiq'a Ka'a *(Dena'ina),*
Cháas' *(Tlingit),* Amaqtuuq *(Iñupiaq)*

Alaska Seafood Marketing Institute

The pink salmon is also known as the "Humpback" or "Humpy" because of the flattened hump which develops on the back of an adult male before spawning. The pink salmon is the smallest of the Pacific salmon found in North America and can grow up to four pounds in weight and measure 20 to 25 inches in length.

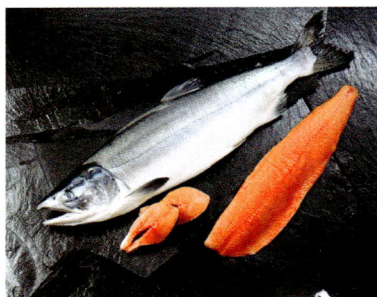

PREPARATION: Pink salmon can be baked, broiled, grilled, fried, steamed, or poached. Pinks can be dried, hung in the heat of summer, because they have less oil than other salmon. They dry with a salty taste, and shrink hard when they dry, like pike. The dried fish can be stored in seal oil.

76

"I took my grandson out in a skiff to catch pinks. We caught 15 fish, and then went house to house to give to elders. At the last elder's house, we gave away the only fish left. After leaving, my grandson asked 'Umma, what are we going to do? My mom needs fish too.' I said we can go fishing tomorrow. This was my grandson's first experience of the 'gift of giving' to others."

– Eleanor McMullen, Port Graham

PINK SALMON NUTRITION INFORMATION

Pink salmon is an excellent source of protein

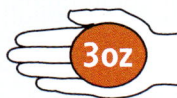

PROTEIN

3oz

MAN   WOMAN

HEART FRIENDLY
- Low in saturated fat
- Low in sodium

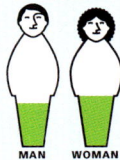

NUTRITION INFORMATION	
Per serving - 3 oz: dried	
Calories	127
Protein	22 g
Carbohydrate	0 g
Fat	4 g
Calories from fat	28 %
Saturated fat	1 g
Dietary Fiber	0
Cholesterol	57 mg
Sodium	73 mg
Vitamin A	116 IU
Vitamin C	0
Iron	1 mg

Red Salmon
Sockeye

NATIVE NAMES:
Sayak *(Yup'ik)*,
Q'uya *(Dena'ina)*, Gaat *(Tlingit)*

Sockeye salmon from Alaska's waters rank among the world's finest seafood. The natural environment provides them with superior flavor, color and texture. Thousands of salmon travel through Alaska's rivers and streams returning to their place of origin to spawn.

Alaska Seafood Marketing Institute

PREPARATION: Red salmon can be baked, broiled, grilled, fried, steamed, or poached.

Red salmon have a distinctive deep-red color that is retained when cooking. Their fat content depends on where they are caught. They are often good for drying. Commercial fishermen refer to these salmon as "money-fish" because they fish for red salmon to make money.

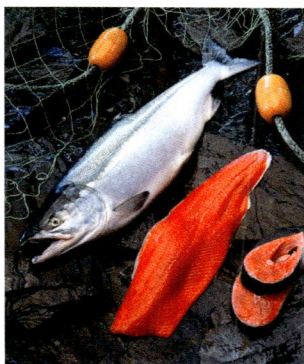

77

RED SALMON NUTRITION INFORMATION

Red salmon is an excellent source of protein and a good source of iron

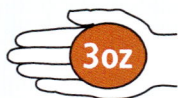

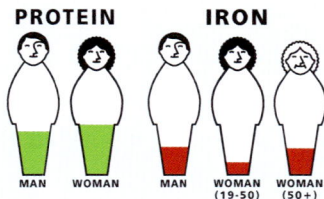

3oz

PROTEIN   **IRON**

MAN WOMAN   MAN WOMAN (19-50) WOMAN (50+)

HEART FRIENDLY
● Low in saturated fat

NUTRITION INFORMATION	
Per serving - 3 oz: canned	
Calories	137
Protein	23 g
Carbohydrate	0
Fat	5 g
Calories from fat	33 %
Saturated fat	1 g
Dietary Fiber	0
Cholesterol	59 mg
Sodium	332 mg
Vitamin A	184 IU
Vitamin C	0
Iron	2 g

Silver Salmon

Coho

NATIVE NAMES: Qakiiyaq *(Yup'ik)*, Nudlegha *(Dena'ina)*, L'ook *(Tlingit)*, Iqalukpik *(Iñupiaq)*

Alaska Seafood Marketing Institute

Silver salmon is one of the most important and frequently used traditional food sources. Also called coho salmon, silver salmon in central and western Alaska are found in coastal waters of Alaska from Dixon Entrance in Southeastern Alaska, as far north as Point Hope, and up the Yukon River to the Alaska-Yukon border. Silver salmon enter spawning river systems from August through November, usually during periods of high water.

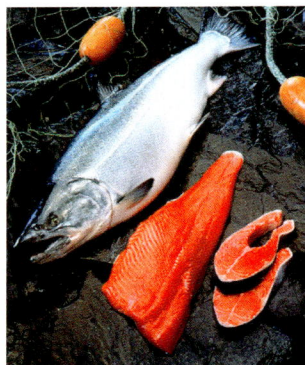

PREPARATION: Silver salmon can be baked, broiled, grilled, fried, steamed, or poached. They have more fat than sockeye salmon, but less than king salmon.

78

"Of all my traditional Native foods, I love dried fish . . . I live next to a stream that is one hundred feet from my house, and I fish there. The fun part of going after fish, whether it's sockeye, dogfish, humpies, coho, or silvers, is being physically active. Being involved in the preparation process--doing the work, getting the wood, hanging the fish to dry, and caring for the fish. You don't just walk away."
— *Lincoln Bean, Kake*

SILVER SALMON NUTRITION INFORMATION

Silver salmon is an excellent source of protein

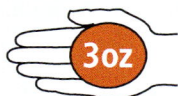

PROTEIN

MAN WOMAN

3oz

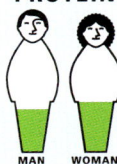

HEART FRIENDLY
- Low in saturated fat
- Low in sodium

NUTRITION INFORMATION	
Per serving - 3 oz: raw	
Calories	123
Protein	19 g
Carbohydrate	1 g
Fat	5 g
Calories from fat	37 %
Saturated fat	1 g
Dietary Fiber	0
Cholesterol	49 mg
Sodium	49 mg
Vitamin A	85 IU
Vitamin C	0
Iron	0

Salmon Eggs

Roe, Salmon Caviar

NATIVE NAMES:
Meluk *(Yup'ik),*
Kaháakw *(Tlingit)*

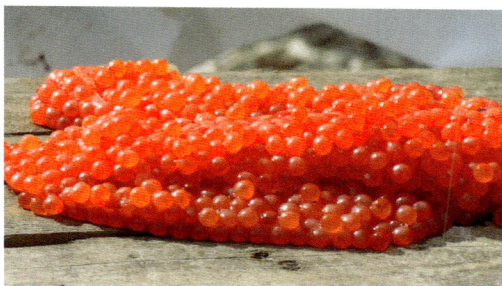

Tanana Chiefs Conference

A by-product of salmon, salmon eggs or roe are a tasty delicacy, and sometimes referred to as "salmon caviar." The eggs are bright orange in color and the size of a small pea.

PREPARATION: Salmon eggs can be boiled with fish, dried, fried, or used as a garnish in other dishes. Salmon eggs become firm and chewy when dried.

Every part of a fish is used, including the roe – dried salmon eggs are a favorite food of Yup'ik elders.

79

SALMON EGGS NUTRITION INFORMATION

Salmon eggs are an excellent source of protein

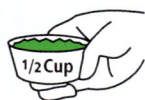

PROTEIN

MAN   WOMAN

1/2 Cup

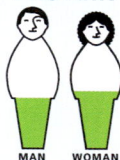

NUTRITION INFORMATION	
Per serving - 1/2 cup: raw	
Calories	212
Protein	25 g
Carbohydrate	2 g
Fat	12 g
Calories from fat	51 %
Saturated fat	2 g
Dietary Fiber	NT*
Cholesterol	147 mg
Sodium	NT*
Vitamin A	0
Vitamin C	NT*
Iron	NT*

*Not Tested

Sea Cucumber

NATIVE NAMES: Yéin *(Tlingit)*,
Yano *(Haida)*

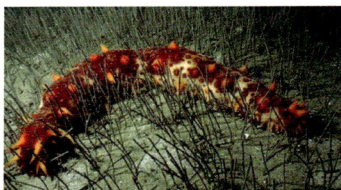

The giant red sea cucumber is
commercially harvested largely
in Southeast Alaska, with a small
amount harvested in Kodiak and Chignik.
The sea cucumber looks like a giant slug
with spiny skin. They can grow up to one and one-half feet in
length, and weigh one pound. They are found at the bottom of
tidal pools. Sea cucumber is typically harvested from early spring
to late fall.

*Alaska Fisheries Science Center,
NOAA Fisheries Service*

PREPARATION: Collect sea cucumbers at extreme low
tide in June through August. Cut off each end. Squeeze out the
insides and wash them clean. Split the sea cucumber lengthwise
and peel off its outer skin, leaving the long white muscles. Sea
cucumber may be: chopped for chowder; chopped and scrambled
in omelettes; dipped in egg, then coated in flour or breadcrumbs
and fried quickly; ground for patties, mixed with flour and egg
batter; and used in chop suey.

*Sea cucumbers were traditionally harvested with spears and long
poles, and then boiled or roasted over a campfire. The Tlingits call
sea cucumbers yein, or "sea sweet potato."*

SEA CUCUMBER NUTRITION INFORMATION

Sea cucmber is an
excellent source of
protein and a good
source of Vitamin A

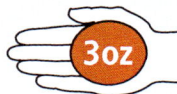

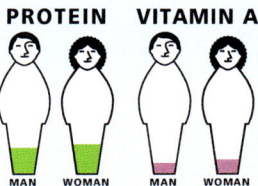

3oz

PROTEIN **VITAMIN A**

MAN WOMAN MAN WOMAN

HEART FRIENDLY
• Fat free

NUTRITION INFORMATION	
Per serving - 3 oz	
Calories	58
Protein	11 g
Carbohydrate	3 g
Fat	0
Calories from fat	0 %
Saturated fat	NT*
Dietary Fiber	NT*
Cholesterol	NT*
Sodium	NT*
Vitamin A	264 IU
Vitamin C	NT*
Iron	1 mg

*Not Tested

Sea Lion

NATIVE NAMES: Apakcuk
(Yup'ik),
Ta'ilk'eghi *(Dena'ina)*,
Taan *(Tlingit)*

Steller sea lions were traditionally a primary source of food for inhabitants of the Aleutian Islands. They are called sea lions because they resemble the lions of Africa and Asia.

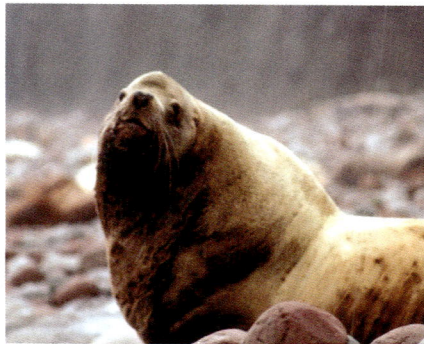

U.S. Fish & Wildlife Service

PREPARATION: Sea lion meat can be cooked in any regular meat dish, stewed, fried, or eaten plain.

"Sea lion was a big deal for people in Kodiak, better meal than seal. My parents always talked about sea lion. Just a few weeks ago, I had a feast of bear, seal and sea lion (served separately) simmered in their own gravy—that's how I like to eat it!"

– *Iver Malutin, Kodiak*

81

SEA LION NUTRITION INFORMATION

Sea lion is an excellent source of protein & iron, and is a good source of Vitamin A

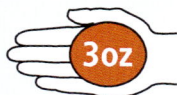

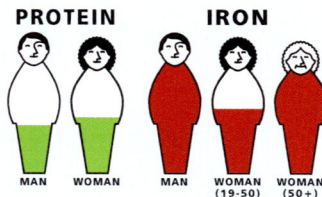

3oz

PROTEIN   IRON

MAN   WOMAN   MAN   WOMAN   WOMAN
                         (19-50)   (50+)

HEART FRIENDLY
• Low in sodium

NUTRITION INFORMATION	
Per serving - 3 oz: meat with fat (raw)	
Calories	160
Protein	20 g
Carbohydrate	2 g
Fat	8 g
Calories from fat	45 %
Saturated fat	2 g
Dietary Fiber	0 g
Cholesterol	53 mg
Sodium	61 mg
Vitamin A	246 IU
Vitamin C	<3 mg
Iron	9 mg

Seal

NATIVE NAMES:
Taqukaq *(Yup'ik)*,
Qutsaghiłʼiy *(Dena'ina)*,
Xʼóon *(Tlingit)*,
Isux̂ *(Unangam Tunuu)*

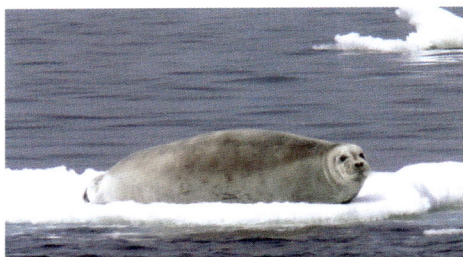

U.S. Fish & Wildlife Service

Seal is a delicacy among Alaska Native people who harvest it year round. Some prefer to hunt seal in the early spring when they are fattest and will render the most seal oil.

PREPARATION: The meat is a dark red-black color. Seal meat can be cooked in any regular meat dish, stewed, fried, or eaten plain. Almost every part of the seal is eaten.

"To prepare fur seal flippers, "lusta," let them ferment in rock salt for a few months. I would see my mom preparing them with other ladies, who would get together and eat the flippers with potatos and seal oil. Lusta is considered a delicacy and is cut to ½ the size of a pinky nail in order for it to digest well in the system."

– Tina Woods

"I was taught to give my first catch of seal to an elder in the community; I remember being reluctant, but did it anyway. The elder said to me, 'God bless you with many more; God bless you with everything.'"

– Dan Karmun, Nome (grew up in Deering)

SEAL NUTRITION INFORMATION

*nutrient data based on ringed seal

Seal is an excellent source of protein & iron, and a good source of Vitamin A

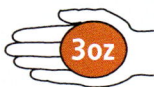

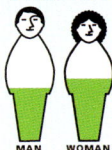

PROTEIN

MAN   WOMAN

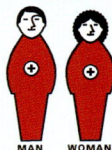

IRON

MAN   WOMAN

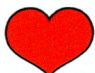

HEART FRIENDLY
● Low in sodium

NUTRITION INFORMATION	
Per serving - 3 oz: raw	
Calories	121
Protein	24 g
Carbohydrate	0
Fat	3 g
Calories from fat	22 %
Saturated fat	1 g
Dietary Fiber	NT*
Cholesterol	76 mg
Sodium	9 mg
Vitamin A	327 IU
Vitamin C	NT*
Iron	17 mg

*Not Tested

82

Seal Oil

NATIVE NAMES: Uquq *(Yup'ik)*,
Qutsaghił'iy Tlegh *(Dena'ina)*,
Misibaaq *(Iñupiaq)*

Seal oil that is properly prepared and stored is sweet and has a clear consistency (milky when frozen). Seal oil uses include: added as a flavor in agutak, fish dishes, and soups; used as a dip; and used as a trade item for other Native foods.

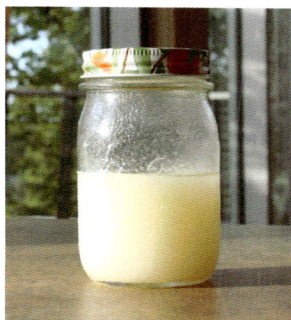

Patricia Bunyan

PREPARATION: Seal oil preparation varies by Alaska region. Seal oil is used for a dip when eating dried meats and fish, potatoes, herring eggs, and can also be used to complement other Native foods.

"I don't feel full until I eat Native food, like a little seal oil at the end of a meal."

— *Elder*

83

SEAL OIL NUTRITION INFORMATION

*nutrient data based on spotted seal oil

Seal oil is a good source of Vitamin A

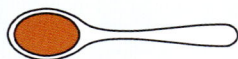

VITAMIN A

MAN   WOMAN

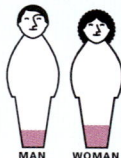

HEART FRIENDLY
- Low in sodium

NUTRITION INFORMATION	
Per serving - 1 tablespoon	
Calories	125
Protein	0
Carbohydrate	0
Fat	15 g
Calories from fat	100 %
Saturated fat	2 g
Dietary Fiber	0
Cholesterol	NT*
Sodium	0
Vitamin A	487 IU
Vitamin C	0
Iron	0
*Not Tested	

Shrimp

NATIVE NAMES: **Cungaralukvak** *(Yup'ik)*,
Ts'enełts'eha *(Dena'ina)*,
S'éex'át *(Tlingit)*, **Igliġaq** *(Iñupiaq)*

There are five varieties of shrimp found in Alaska's North Pacific waters: coon-stripe, humpy, pink, side-stripe, and spot. Larger shrimp are known as prawns and smaller sized as cocktail shrimp. Pink shrimp is the largest harvest in Alaska. Light weight pots are used to catch shrimp for personal use.

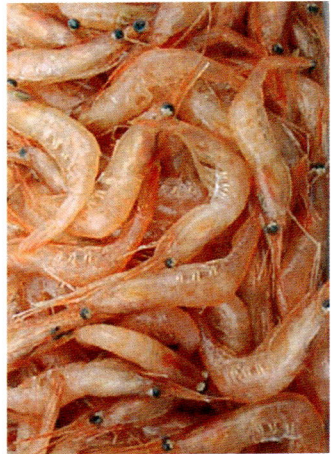

Alaska Fisheries Science Center, NOAA Fisheries Service

PREPARATION: Shrimp can be prepared many different ways: simmered, baked, boiled, fried, in casseroles, salads, and sauces.

84

Traditionally, shrimp were enjoyed whenever a quantity was found in a sea mammal's stomach.

SHRIMP NUTRITION INFORMATION

*nutrient data based on mixed species

Shrimp is an excellent source of protein and a good source of iron

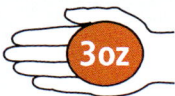

3oz

PROTEIN   **IRON**

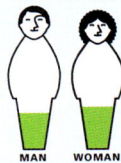
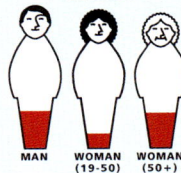

MAN   WOMAN   MAN   WOMAN (19-50)   WOMAN (50+)

HEART FRIENDLY
- Low in fat
- Saturated fat free

NUTRITION INFORMATION	
Per serving - 3 oz: cooked	
Calories	84
Protein	18 g
Carbohydrate	0
Fat	1 g
Calories from fat	11 %
Saturated fat	0
Dietary Fiber	0
Cholesterol	166 mg
Sodium	190 mg
Vitamin A	191 IU
Vitamin C	2 mg
Iron	3 mg

Sticklebacks
Needlefish

NATIVE NAMES: Quarruuk *(Yup'ik)*, Dgheyay *(Dena'ina)*, Took *(Tlingit)*

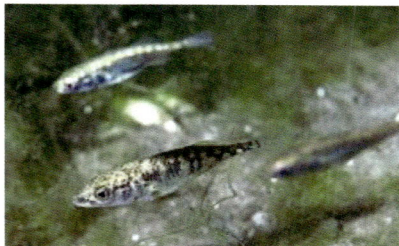

Sticklebacks are a small, slender fish, greenish in color, that grows to 4 inches in length. Sticklebacks have a row of nine short spines on their back in front of their dorsal fin. Sticklebacks are harvested in great quantities in small streams and waterways, and can be found in Southern and Western Alaska.

PREPARATION: Sticklebacks are usually eaten raw while the fish is still alive. The fish head is swallowed first to prevent its spiny back from sticking to the throat.

The Dena'ina of Cook Inlet would survive on sticklebacks until the salmon began to run.

85

STICKLEBACK NUTRITION INFORMATION

Sticklebacks are an excellent source of Vitamin A, and a good source of protein

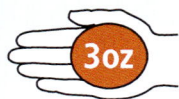

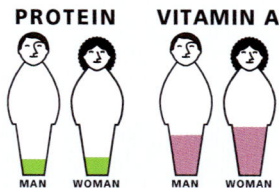

3oz

PROTEIN

VITAMIN A

MAN WOMAN MAN WOMAN

NUTRITION INFORMATION	
Per serving - 3 oz	
Calories	86
Protein	8 g
Carbohydrate	1 g
Fat	5 g
Calories from fat	52 %
Saturated fat	NT*
Dietary Fiber	NT*
Cholesterol	NT*
Sodium	NT*
Vitamin A	1046 IU
Vitamin C	0
Iron	5 mg
*Not Tested	

Trout

NATIVE NAMES:
Anerrluaq *(Yup'ik),*
Tsagela *(Dena'ina),* **Yaa**
(Tlingit)

There are many species of trout in Alaska, including sea trout, Dolly Varden, and Arctic char. They are found in lakes, streams and in the sea.

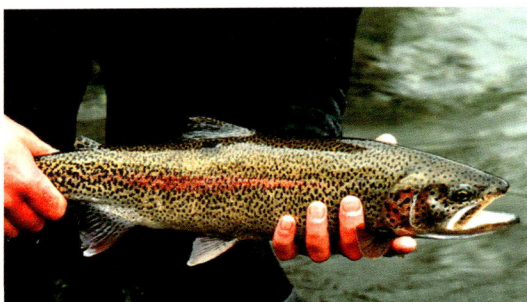

U.S. Fish & Wildlife Service

PREPARATION: Trout can be roasted or eaten frozen. They may also be boiled, baked, fried, or made into trout soup. Trout livers can be prepared with blueberries and eaten at any meal or for dessert. Trout can be hard to dry when they are fat. They can be half-dried for one to four days, then boiled and eaten with seal oil. Trout may also be stored pickled with blueberries.

86

Trout were traditionally pickled with sourdock in Northwestern Alaska, which caused their bones to soften and become edible.

TROUT NUTRITION INFORMATION

*nutrient data based on wild rainbow trout

Trout is an excellent source of protein

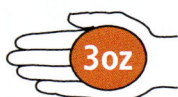

3oz

PROTEIN

MAN   WOMAN

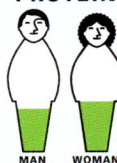

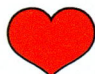

HEART FRIENDLY
- Low in saturated fat
- Low in sodium

NUTRITION INFORMATION	
Per serving - 3 oz: cooked	
Calories	128
Protein	19 g
Carbohydrate	0
Fat	5 g
Calories from fat	35 %
Saturated fat	1 g
Dietary Fiber	0
Cholesterol	59 mg
Sodium	48 mg
Vitamin A	42 IU
Vitamin C	2 mg
Iron	0

Walrus

NATIVE NAMES: Asveq *(Yup'ik)*, Hnihik'ghiłtsatl'i *(Dena'ina)*, Kooléix'waa *(Tlingit)*, Aiviq *(Iñupiaq)*

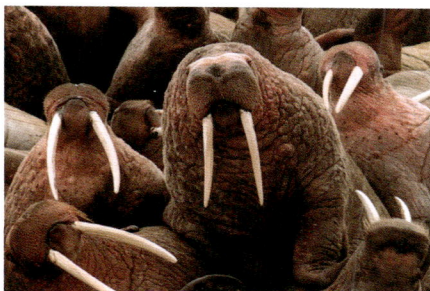

Walruses prefer to inhabit shallow water areas, close to ice or land. They are harvested from villages near the coast of the Bering Strait and

U.S. Fish & Wildlife Service

from St. Lawrence Island, King Island, and Little Diomede Island. Adult females can weigh up to 2,000 pounds, with males weighing more than 4,000 pounds. There are many traditional uses of walrus: the use of the meat for food, the skins for making boat and house covers, the intestines are eaten and were used for rain coats, the bones for tools, the stomach for containers and drums, the hide for clothing and house covers, the meat for dog food, the fresh hide for the preservation of other foods and the ivory for useful and decorative implements.

PREPARATION: Walrus meat can be baked, boiled, or fried, with the meat slow cooked to an internal temperature of 185°F to kill any parasites. Walrus meat can be cut into thin steaks and tenderized.

Walrus is a prized subsistence food for Alaska Native people living in Alaska's coastal communities. A good walrus harvest can provide a village with enough meat for a year.

87

WALRUS NUTRITION INFORMATION

Walrus is an excellent source of protein & iron

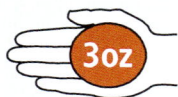

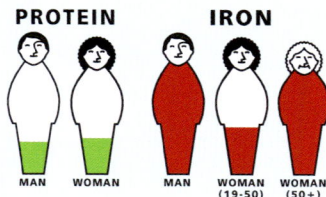

3oz

PROTEIN

MAN WOMAN

IRON

MAN WOMAN (19-50) WOMAN (50+)

NUTRITION INFORMATION	
Per serving - 3 oz: raw	
Calories	169
Protein	16 g
Carbohydrate	0
Fat	12 g
Calories from fat	64 %
Saturated fat	2 g
Dietary Fiber	NT*
Cholesterol	68 mg
Sodium	NT*
Vitamin A	144 IU
Vitamin C	NT*
Iron	8 mg

*Not Tested

Whitefish

Broad, Humpback, Pygmy, Round, Least Cisco, Bering Cisco, Arctic Cisco, Sheefish

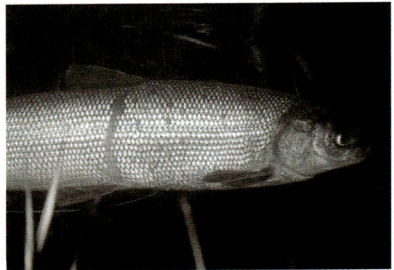

Thomas C. Kline, Jr.

NATIVE NAMES: Cavirrutnaq *(Yup'ik),* Łih *(Dena'ina),* Savigunnaq - *Round (Iñupiaq),* Aanaakliq - *Broad (Iñupiaq),* Pikuktuuq - *Humpback (Iñupiaq)*

Whitefish are the most abundant group of fish north of the Alaska Range, inhabiting almost every type of river or freshwater habitat in Alaska. In Northwest Alaska, part of a caribou's shoulder blade bone was traditionally used to scale whitefish. The fish are caught in traps from break up until after freeze up.

PREPARATION: Whitefish have delicious, white, flaky, mild tasting flesh. They can be eaten in a wide variety of ways depending on how fat they are: raw, half dried, and dried; cooked rare or well done; cooked in most fish recipes, roasted over the fire; eaten frozen, fermented, or boiled whitefish is also used in agutak.

Koyukon people held a small ceremony when the first whitefish was taken in the spring. They had survived another winter—cause enough for celebration—and now the secure abundance of summer was just ahead.

WHITEFISH NUTRITION INFORMATION

Whitefish is an excellent source of protein & Vitamin A

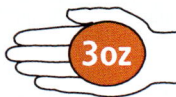

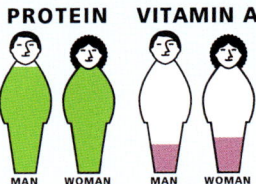

PROTEIN   **VITAMIN A**

3oz

NUTRITION INFORMATION	
Per serving - 3 oz: dried	
Calories	315
Protein	53 g
Carbohydrate	0
Fat	11 g
Calories from fat	31 %
Saturated fat	2 g
Dietary Fiber	0
Cholesterol	226 mg
Sodium	170 mg
Vitamin A	620 IU
Vitamin C	0
Iron	3 mg

Whitefish Eggs

NATIVE NAMES: Q'in *(Dena'ina)*

Whitefish eggs are usually harvested by jigging in the open river or by ice fishing in the winter. Salmon eggs are used to lure the whitefish, which usually end up stealing the eggs from the "J" hook. You need eggs to get their eggs.

PREPARATION: Cook whitefish eggs by blanching them in simmering water. Traditionally they were generally eaten raw, right after a female whitefish was caught. They are said to slip right down your throat.

"Only catch enough fish to last you through the winter. Use or preserve every part of the fish that is edible. Fish are easy to spoil, especially the whitefish, so take care of the fish as soon as they are caught. If we are lazy and idle, food won't come to us."

– Henry Frank

89

"When I was five years old, I remember how a neighboring village used to catch whitefish using a 'fish fence' made out of driftwood and willow trees. Before freeze up, and depending on the width of the river, the wood and trees were placed in the river with several one to two feet openings to create passage ways for the fish. A dip net was then used to catch the fish passing through the openings. Sadly, they don't fish this way anymore. But, I always remember watching other people catching the fish."

– Levi Brink, Kasigluk

WHITEFISH EGG NUTRITION INFORMATION

Whitefish eggs are an excellent source of protein, and a good source of Vitamin C

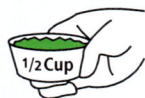

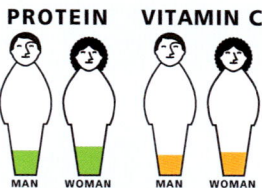

1/2 Cup

PROTEIN **VITAMIN C**

MAN WOMAN MAN WOMAN

HEART FRIENDLY
• Low in sodium

NUTRITION INFORMATION	
Per serving - 1/2 cup: raw	
Calories	88
Protein	12 g
Carbohydrate	4 g
Fat	2 g
Calories from fat	20 %
Saturated fat	0
Dietary Fiber	0
Cholesterol	373 mg
Sodium	136 mg
Vitamin A	257 IU
Vitamin C	10 mg
Iron	5 mg

Whale

Beluga, Bowhead

NATIVE NAMES:
Arveq *(Yup'ik)*,
Tałin *(Dena'ina)*,
Yáay *(Tlingit)*, Qilalugaq/
Sisuaq - *Beluga (Iñupiaq)*
Aġviq - *Bowhead (Iñupiaq)*

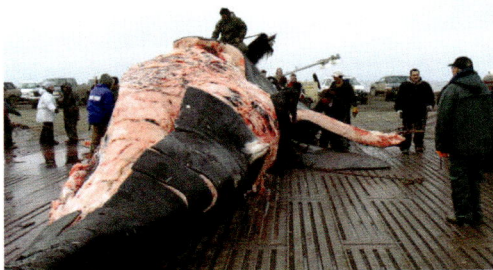

Donald Zanoff

For centuries whales were hunted for their valuable oil and very fine grained meat. Alaska Native people in the North continue to harvest whales as a source of food and fuel, as they have traditionally done for thousands of years.

PREPARATION: Whale meat can be prepared by pan-broiling the square steaks and serving them sizzling hot. Whale meat is also excellent for soup stock, stews, roasts, and curries. Another way to enjoy whale is to eat the muktuk (the outer covering of the whale), which is traditionally eaten raw or cooked.

90

September brings whaling season to Kaktovik, a village-wide activity. Women prepare food to send out with the whaling crews and wait on the beach for the crews to return with a whale. The day after the whale is beached, everyone goes to the captain's house to eat whale meat and muktuk. They spend the whole day visiting and eating and then take some of the leftover whale meat home with them.

– Frances Lampe, Kaktovik

WHALE NUTRITION INFORMATION

Whale is an excellent source of protein & iron

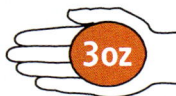

PROTEIN

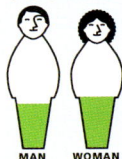

MAN   WOMAN

IRON

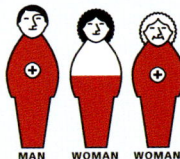

MAN   WOMAN (19-50)   WOMAN (50+)

HEART FRIENDLY
● Lean
● Low in sodium

NUTRITION INFORMATION	
Per serving - 3 oz: cooked	
Calories	115
Protein	22 g
Carbohydrate	0
Fat	6 g
Calories from fat	48 %
Saturated fat	1 g
Dietary Fiber	0
Cholesterol	24 mg
Sodium	85 mg
Vitamin A	280 IU
Vitamin C	6 mg
Iron	12 mg

"It has been believed by the Native people for many years that animals, just like human beings, have spirits. The belief has always been there that you must treat the animals with respect. I think it has been traditional for every tribe that ever existed in the world to try not to make the animals that you hunt for food suffer. If you are going to kill an animal, make it clean and quick….you do not waste them. You do not play with them. There was a belief that if you played with them, you are insulting the animals, birds and fish. And a lot of times they think the spirits of those animals, birds and fish will turn around and tell the other animals: 'Don't go to that person. He hasn't any respect for us.' And that person, the hunter, will not be able to catch anything."

— *Chuck Hunt (born near Kotlik, worked as a U.S. Fish and Wildlife translator in Bethel*

"When I was 10 years old, and living in Kwigillnok, my father wanted me to go hunting with him and retrieve ducks after he shot them. My mother warned me not to play with the ducks if they were just injured. She said if I did, my father wouldn't get any more ducks that day. I began retrieving the ducks after my father shot them, sloshing through the mud and water. When I found one that was only injured, I played with it, not heeding my mother's warning. My father didn't get any more ducks that day."

— *Nina M. Heavener, Clarks Point*

"When I think of plants...and of all living things;
I remember being told and learning about how everything
works together and interacts with one another. When
gathering, I notice that plants, medicinal and edible, have
complex relationships. It is the whole of the plant and
its place in the environment that determines the plant's
potency and compatibilty with others."

– Gloria Simeon, Bethel

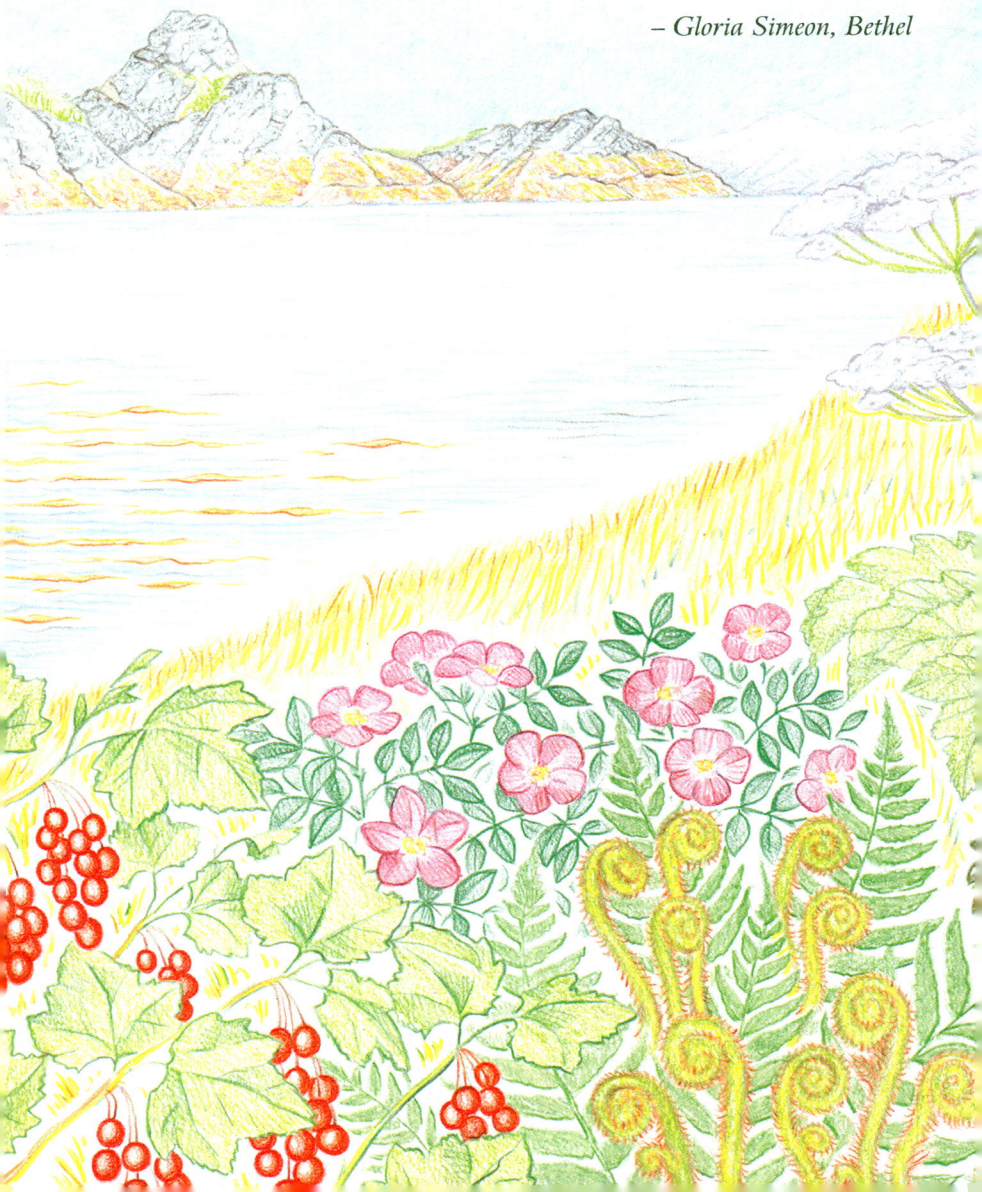

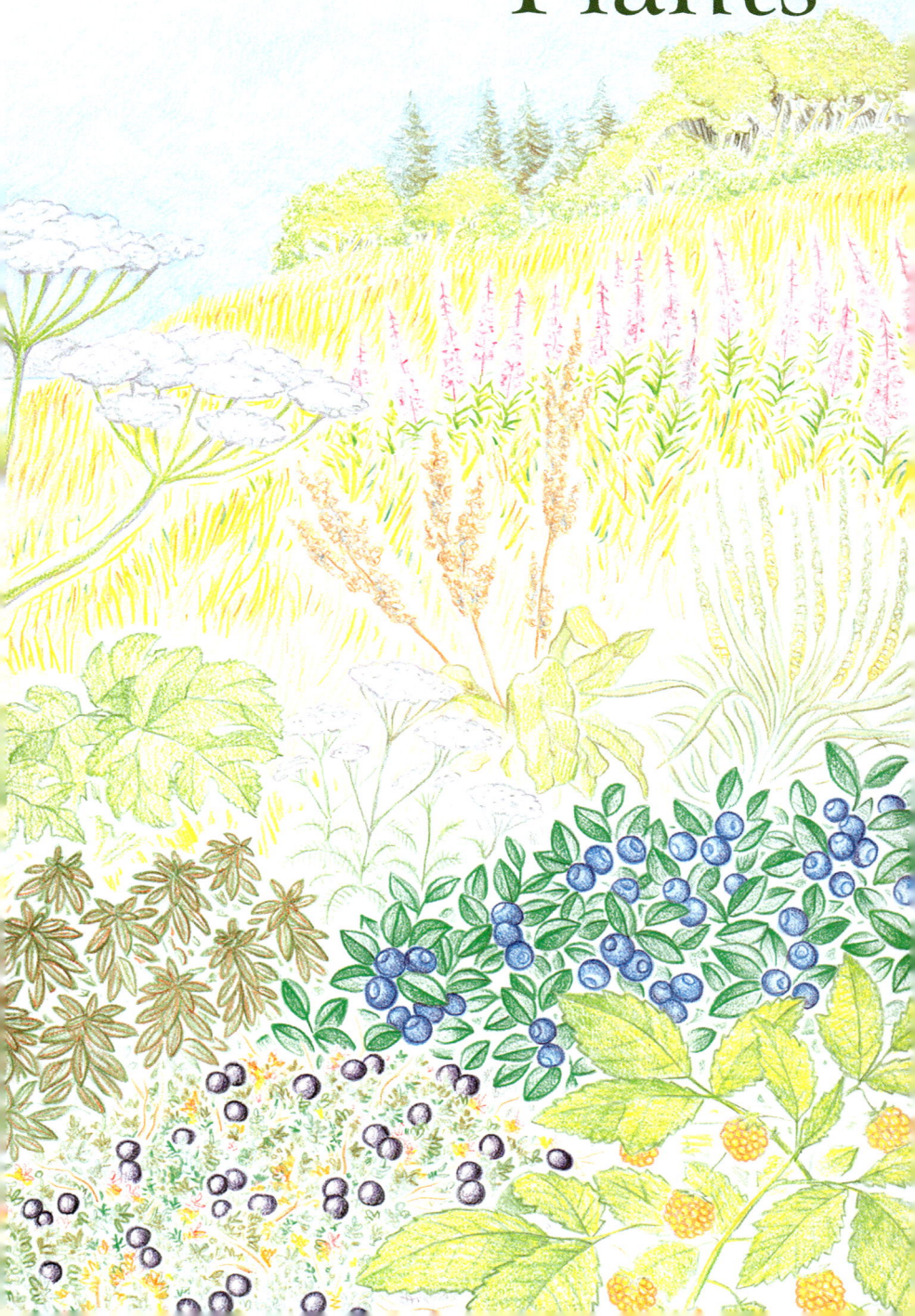

Plants

Beach Asparagus

Sea Asparagus,
Pickleweed

NATIVE NAMES:
It'garralek *(Yup'ik),*
Su<u>k</u>káadzi *(Tlingit)*

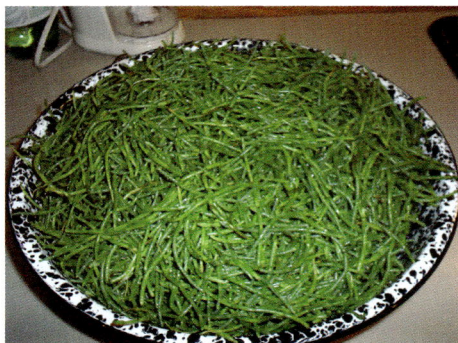

Libby Watanabe

Similar to asparagus and green beans, beach asparagus are the small, fleshy stems and branches of salty seacoast plants. A young plant looks like a tiny cactus, or branching coral with reddish tips. It is found on the beaches and bays of Southeastern Alaska, and is harvested in late spring throughout the summer. If picked later, after the plant has flowered, the beach asparagus has a "woody" taste.

94

PREPARATION: Beach asparagus are crisp and tender, and can be eaten raw. As summer moves on, they become a little crunchier and they may be briefly boiled. Older, tougher beach asparagus can be steamed along with mussels, clams or crabs. Their sea-breeze scent enhances the fresh aroma of the shellfish sharing the pot.

"They told me to eat kale when I was getting cancer treatment. I don't even know what kale is. I wanted sea asparagus."
— *Ethel Lund, Juneau*

BEACH ASPARAGUS NUTRITION INFORMATION

Beach asparagus is an excellent source of Vitamin A

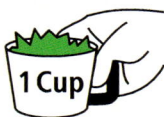

VITAMIN A

1 Cup

HEART FRIENDLY
- Fat free • Low calorie
- Very low in sodium

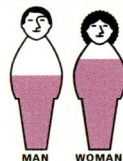

NUTRITION INFORMATION	
Per serving - 1 cup: raw	
Calories	15
Protein	1 g
Carbohydrate	2 g
Fat	0
Calories from fat	0 %
Saturated fat	0
Dietary Fiber	NT*
Cholesterol	NT*
Sodium	23 mg
Vitamin A	1057 IU
Vitamin C	1 mg
Iron	0

*Not Tested

Blueberry

NATIVE NAMES: Curaq *(Yup'ik)*,
Kanat'a *(Tlingit)*,
Uĝiidgin - *bog blueberry (Unangam Tunuu)*, Asiaq *(Iñupiaq)*

ANTHC

Blueberries are found in wooded areas, along waterways, and on the tundra. They can be eaten fresh or frozen. Wild blueberries are very rich in vitamins. A recent study showed that Alaska wild blueberries are even more nutrient rich than wild blueberries in the Lower 48 states.

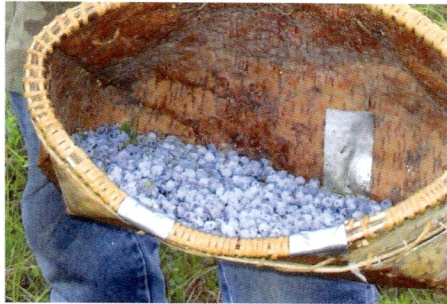

PREPARATION: The Alaskan lowbush blueberry has a tart, fresh flavor and may be used in pies, muffins, and puddings. It may be eaten raw or preserved in sauce, jam, jelly and relish.

In earlier days as barrels of blueberries would freeze, the expanding ice crystals would push up and spill some of the blueberry juice out. It would drip down the side of the barrels and freeze like candle wax. One woman remembers looking forward to picking off those frozen bumps to eat. "They tasted so good, but sometimes they were kind of strong."

95

BLUEBERRIES NUTRITION INFORMATION

Blueberries are an excellent source of Vitamin C, and a good source of fiber

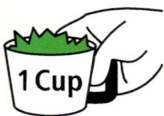

FIBER   **VITAMIN C**

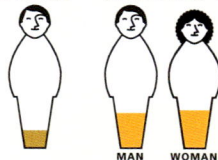

MAN   WOMAN

1 Cup

HEART FRIENDLY
- Low in fat
- Very low in sodium

NUTRITION INFORMATION	
Per serving - 1 cup: raw	
Calories	88
Protein	2 g
Carbohydrate	18 g
Fat	1 g
Calories from fat	11 %
Saturated fat	NT*
Dietary Fiber	4 g
Cholesterol	NT*
Sodium	9 mg
Vitamin A	167 IU
Vitamin C	26.5 mg
Iron	1 mg

*Not Tested

Cloudberry
Low Bush Salmonberry

NATIVE NAMES: Atsalugpiaq *(Yup'ik)*,
Néx̱'w *(Tlingit)*, Aqpik *(Iñupiaq)*,
Algnan *(Unangam Tunuu)*

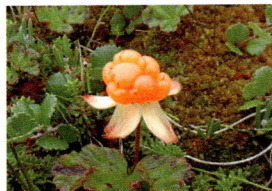

The low bush salmonberry is found mainly in Northern and Western Alaska in bogs, tundra, and open forest areas. Its fruit is ready for harvesting in mid to late fall. When ripe, it has a beautiful golden color. Each low-growing plant bears a single berry, best picked by hand.

PREPARATION: Low bush salmonberries can be prepared in pies, jellies and syrups. Traditionally, they are eaten with sugar and seal oil after a meal. They are best stored frozen, or preserved with other foods, such as blackberries, nagoonberries or sour dock leaves.

96

When a few hard (unripe) salmonberries are mixed with ripe berries, the ones picked too early will turn black and be no good. Stories warning of picking salmonberries too early were often told to teach children, newcomers and greedy people when to pick salmonberries. This would ensure that some berries were left behind for late pickers, or to be given back to the earth for the next season.

CLOUDBERRIES NUTRITION INFORMATION

Cloudberries are an excellent source of Vitamin C, and a good source of Vitamin A

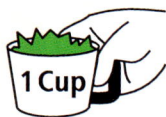

1 Cup

VITAMIN A

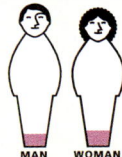

MAN   WOMAN

VITAMIN C

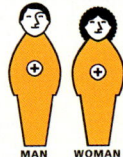

MAN   WOMAN

HEART FRIENDLY
● Low in fat

NUTRITION INFORMATION	
Per serving - 1 cup: raw	
Calories	76
Protein	4 g
Carbohydrate	13 g
Fat	1 g
Calories from fat	14 %
Saturated fat	NT*
Dietary Fiber	NT*
Cholesterol	NT*
Sodium	NT*
Vitamin A	315 IU
Vitamin C	237 mg
Iron	1 mg

*Not Tested

Low Bush Cranberry

Lingonberry

NATIVE NAMES: Kavirliq *(Yup'ik)*,
Dáxw *(Tlingit)*, Kiikan *(Unangam
Tunuu - Eastern dialect)*,
Tuyangis *(UT - Atka dialect)*,
Kimmigeaq *(Iñupiaq)*

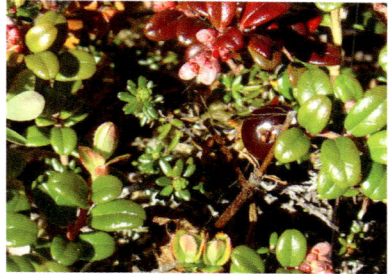

Alaska Plant Materials Center

Low bush cranberries can be picked almost year round. By the end of August some will be ripe enough to cook up for sauce or jam. The full flavor of low bush cranberries does not develop until after the first frost. Unpicked berries remain under the snow all winter and are good to eat frozen, or ready to pick in the spring when the snow melts.

PREPARATION: Low bush cranberries can be eaten in pies, jams, syrups, or by themselves. Low bush cranberries are very tangy when eaten raw, and are often sweetened and cooked. They can be made into cranberry sauce or used in akutaq. Traditionally, they are mixed with meat and fat. To preserve the cranberries, they can be frozen or dried.

The Dena'ina say that the cranberry is more sustaining than any other berry. The Iñupiaq stored cranberries in a qallivik, a special long birch basket with a lid sewn on it, which they kept in a ground pit or propped up in a tree for safe keeping.

97

LOW BUSH CRANBERRIES NUTRITION INFORMATION

Low bush cranberries are an excellent source of Vitamin C

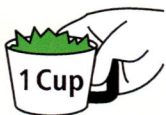

1 Cup

VITAMIN C

MAN   WOMAN

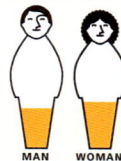

HEART FRIENDLY
• Low in fat

NUTRITION INFORMATION	
Per serving - 1 cup: raw	
Calories	82
Protein	1 g
Carbohydrate	18 g
Fat	1 g
Calories from fat	8 %
Saturated fat	NT*
Dietary Fiber	NT*
Cholesterol	NT*
Sodium	NT*
Vitamin A	135 IU
Vitamin C	32 mg
Iron	1 mg
*Not Tested	

Crowberry
Blackberry, Mossberry

NATIVE NAMES: **Kavlakuaraq** *(Yup'ik),*
Paungaq *(Iñupiaq),*
Qaayun *(Unangam Tunuu - Eastern dialect),*
Aangsus *(Unangam Tunuu - Atka dialect)*

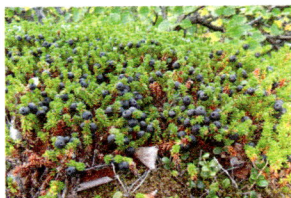

Crowberries grow on low dense mats which cover the ground. They bloom very early in the spring, yet they are the last berry to ripen. The best time to harvest crowberries is just before the first frost when the berries are of maximum size, sweetness and firmness. Crowberries get softer and sweeter after each freeze. Pick the big ones and let the smaller ones keep growing. Return to the same area later to pick them when ripe.

PREPARATION: The flavor of the crowberries can be brought out by cooking. The mild sweet berry is enjoyed eaten with sugar and milk, in agutak, cereal, or seal oil. To preserve them, the berries have traditionally been stored in seal oil, or mixed with other berries and frozen. The Iñupiaq people mix their berries with fish livers.

"When you are very thirsty, look for crowberries; they satisfy your thirst quickly."

98

CROWBERRY NUTRITION INFORMATION

Crowberries are an excellent source of fiber

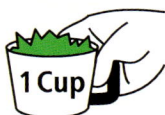

1 Cup

FIBER

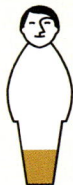

HEART FRIENDLY
- Low in fat
- Very low in sodium

NUTRITION INFORMATION	
Per serving - 1 cup: raw	
Calories	75
Protein	1 g
Carbohydrate	14 g
Fat	1 g
Calories from fat	18 %
Saturated fat	NT*
Dietary Fiber	5 g
Cholesterol	NT*
Sodium	4 mg
Vitamin A	67 IU
Vitamin C	7 mg
Iron	0

*Not Tested

Eskimo Potato

NATIVE NAMES: Marallaq or Masru *(Yup'ik)*, Masu *(Iñupiaq)*

The Eskimo potato is a tall plant. It grows up to two feet tall, and has long flower stalks with many small narrow light pink to purple pea-shaped flowers. It is dug up just before freeze-up, after the first hard frost, and in the spring time after the ground thaws.

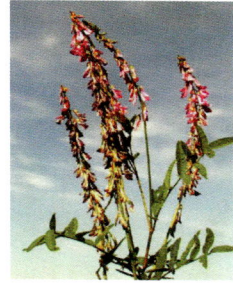

Alaska Plant Materials Center

CAUTION: There are similar looking plants, such as the wild sweet pea, that are poisonous. It is important to be positive that you are harvesting the Eskimo potato.

PREPARATION: Eskimo potatoes can be eaten raw, boiled, baked, or fried. The Dena'ina Athabascans boil the roots with berries and add bear fat; fry the root in fat; put it in hot water for a drink; or eat it raw with moose grease.

A basket of roots might be traded for a fur blanket or an undisclosed amount of dry fish. In dire times these roots would be gathered in the winter and they were known for saving many lives.

99

"The Eskimo potato is a root that can be picked in the spring or fall. Cut in bite size pieces and freeze; soak in seal oil; mix with other wild plants (willow leaves, wild celery) and carrots. Add dried fish, muktuk (whale blubber) or black meat (dried seal meat). Chill for a few hours to allow the flavors to mix. The salad makes a wonderful trail mix for an instant meal or snack." – Emily Hughes, Teller

ESKIMO POTATO NUTRITION INFORMATION

*Nutrient data based on regular potato

Eskimo potato is a good source of protein and Vitamin C

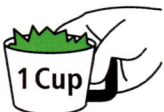

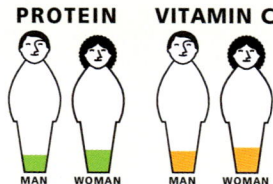

PROTEIN

VITAMIN C

MAN WOMAN   MAN WOMAN

1 Cup

NUTRITION INFORMATION	
Per serving - 1 cup: raw	
Calories	202
Protein	9 g
Carbohydrate	34 g
Fat	4 g
Calories from fat	18 %
Saturated fat	NT*
Dietary Fiber	NT*
Cholesterol	NT*
Sodium	NT*
Vitamin A	24 IU
Vitamin C	17 mg
Iron	NT*

*Not Tested

Fiddlehead Fern

NATIVE NAMES: Cetuguar *(Yup'ik)*, K'wál<u>x</u> *(Tlingit)*

Fiddlehead ferns are also known as the "trailing wood" fern. Fiddleheads are the coiled edible spring growth of ferns. They can be found from the Brooks Range southward toward the Aleutian Islands, and on the Alaska Panhandle. To harvest them, pick the tightly coiled fiddleheads in early spring. Fiddlehead fern rootstock can be harvested in early spring or fall.

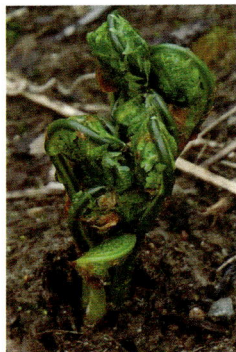

Alaska Plant Materials Center

CAUTION: Pick fiddleheads only when they are young and tightly coiled, as the mature ferns are toxic.

PREPARATION: Fiddleheads should always be cooked before eating. The tighter the head the tastier it will be. Fiddleheads can be prepared by steaming, boiling, or baking. Before cooking fiddleheads, rub off the bitter brown chaff on the stalks and rinse them with water.

100

"In the early spring one year, the people ran out of food. They divided into two groups, one moving into the higher country to dig ferns, and the other to the salt water to dig clams. Those people who lived on ferns received back their strength and gained weight, while those that lived on clams barely survived."

– Tanaina Plantlore

FIDDLEHEAD FERN NUTRITION INFORMATION

Fiddlehead ferns are an excellent source of fiber and Vitamin A, and a good source of Vitamin C

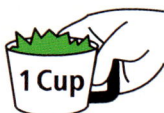

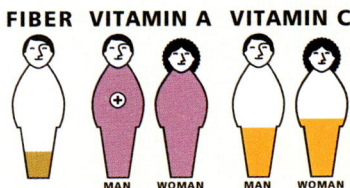

FIBER VITAMIN A VITAMIN C

MAN WOMAN MAN WOMAN

1 Cup

HEART FRIENDLY
- Low in fat
- Very low in sodium

NUTRITION INFORMATION	
Per serving - 1 cup: raw	
Calories	51
Protein	7 g
Carbohydrate	8 g
Fat	1 g
Calories from fat	11 %
Saturated fat	NT*
Dietary Fiber	6 g
Cholesterol	0
Sodium	2 mg
Vitamin A	5426 IU
Vitamin C	40 mg
Iron	2 mg

*Not Tested

Fireweed
Wild Asparagus, Wild Herb

NATIVE NAMES: Ciilqaaq *(Yup'ik)*,
Lóol *(Tlingit)*, Cillqaqtaq *(Alutiiq)*,
Pamiqtaq *(Iñupiaq)*,
Chikayaasix̂ *(Unangam Tunuu - Atka dialect)*

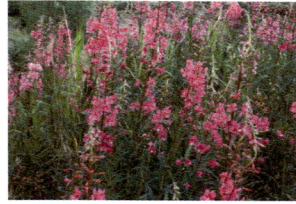

U.S. Fish & Wildlife Service

Fireweed is common throughout Alaska, from the Arctic to the Kenai Peninsula. Traditionally, all parts of this plant have been eaten in a variety of different ways. Fireweed grows best on burned-over land or disturbed soil, along river banks and where people live. Fireweed is ready to pick when the stem is violet colored, the leaves are dark purple, and they are 2 to 4 inches tall. The best time to pick fireweed is in the spring. The plant becomes tough and bitter tasting as it ages.

PREPARATION: Fireweed flowers and leaves are used in salads, soups, casseroles, teas, jams, and honey. Stems and shoots can be boiled, steamed and covered with a cream sauce like asparagus. Fireweed shoots can be bundled and hung to dry for a few days. Wilted fireweed can be preserved in seal oil.

101

"When the fireweed blossoms reach the tip of the stalk, summer is over."

"In Southeast Alaska, the Haida have traditionally gathered tall stems in spring and eaten them at festivals by splitting each shoot lengthwise with the thumb and sprinkling each piece with sugar. Then they pull pieces several inches long through their teeth, scraping off the tender inner part. The remaining fibrous part is twisted into twine for fish nets."

– Alaska Geographic

FIREWEED NUTRITION INFORMATION

Fireweed is an excellent source of Vitamins A & C, and a good source of fiber

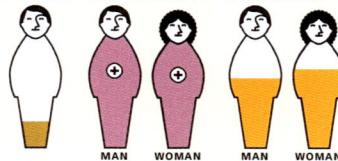

FIBER   VITAMIN A   VITAMIN C

MAN   WOMAN   MAN   WOMAN

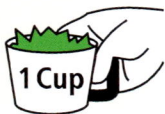

1 Cup

HEART FRIENDLY
• Fat free
• Very low in sodium

NUTRITION INFORMATION	
Per serving - 1 cup: raw	
Calories	24
Protein	2 g
Carbohydrate	3 g
Fat	0
Calories from fat	0 %
Saturated fat	NT*
Dietary Fiber	3 g
Cholesterol	NT*
Sodium	28 mg
Vitamin A	3146 IU
Vitamin C	55 mg
Iron	1 mg

*Not Tested

Goosetongue
Seaside Plantain

NATIVE NAMES: Nutaqitlila *(Dena'ina)*, Suktéitl *(Tlingit)*

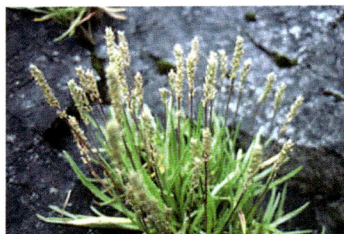

Goosetongue is a popular seaside green found in the coastal and salt marsh areas of Southeast Alaska, the

Scott Brylinsky

Aleutian Islands, and the Seward Peninsula. They have long, thick roots and thick, fleshy leaves and are best harvested from spring to early summer.

CAUTION: The arrow grass plant, which has toxic leaves, closely resembles goosetongue. It is important to be positive that you are harvesting goosetongue.

PREPARATION: Goosetongue can be eaten raw, steamed, blanched, frozen or canned. It tastes great right off the beach, lightly steamed, sautéed, or added to salads, casseroles, and stir-fried dishes.

102

Some Dena'ina say that people learned the use of goosetongue as food from Russians, which may be true. A significant number of Dena'ina people recall Dena'ina names for useful plants, but cannot recall a name for goosetongue.

GOOSETONGUE NUTRITION INFORMATION*

*Nutrient data based on Alaska wild greens

Goosetongue is an excellent source of Vitamins A & C, & a good source of fiber & iron

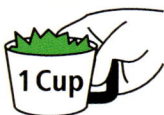

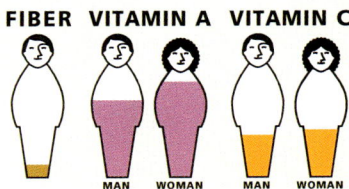

1 Cup

FIBER VITAMIN A VITAMIN C

MAN WOMAN MAN WOMAN

HEART FRIENDLY
- Low in fat
- Low calorie
- Very low in sodium

NUTRITION INFORMATION	
Per serving - 1 cup: cooked	
Calories	25
Protein	2 g
Carbohydrate	4 g
Fat	1 g
Calories from fat	29 %
Saturated fat	0 g
Dietary Fiber	3 g
Cholesterol	0 mg
Sodium	4 mg
Vitamin A	2026 IU
Vitamin C	33 mg
Iron	3 mg

Mouse Food (Roots)
Mouse Caches

NATIVE NAMES: **Anlleq** *(Yup'ik)*,
Nivi *(Iñupiaq)*

Mouse caches provide an easy way to gather roots such as Eskimo potato, or masru. The mouse caches are located by searching for soft spots in the tundra. Once found, the top layer of the ground is gently lifted, and using gloves, the mouse cache is felt out for roots. Only the larger roots are taken, leaving the smaller pieces for the mouse to survive. The cache is carefully repaired by covering with twigs, or grass if available.

PREPARATION: The roots taken from the mouse cache are first cleaned by removing any non-edible roots. They can be eaten raw, boiled, baked, or fried.

The Yup'ik people have passed down from generation to generation that one needs to show respect for the food found in mouse caches. They take only the largest roots and return the smaller ones. In doing this, the mouse will still have food and will not starve and die, and will return the following year to gather more roots. The Iñupiaq add a small repayment like dried fish to thank the mouse for their hard work.

103

MOUSE FOOD NUTRITION INFORMATION

Mouse food is an excellent source of Vitamin C

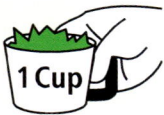

VITAMIN C

MAN   WOMAN

1 Cup

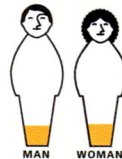

HEART FRIENDLY
• Fat free

NUTRITION INFORMATION	
Per serving - 1 cup	
Calories	89
Protein	4 g
Carbohydrate	18 g
Fat	0
Calories from fat	0 %
Saturated fat	NT*
Dietary Fiber	NT*
Cholesterol	NT*
Sodium	NT*
Vitamin A	NT*
Vitamin C	18 mg
Iron	NT*

*Not Tested

Nettles
Stinging Nettle, Burning Nettle, Indian Spinach

NATIVE NAMES:
Qatlinaq *(Yup'ik),*
T'óok' *(Tlingit)*

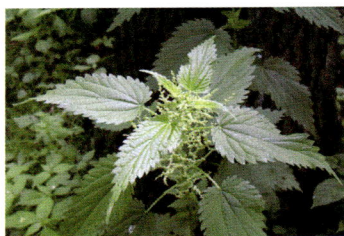

Nettles are found in disturbed and damp soils along stream banks, hillsides and slopes from the Interior to Southeast Alaska. Its leaves have teeth like edges, with the leaf tip pointed. Nettle leaves alternate along the stem. Care needs to be taken in handling the plant. Use gloves as nettle has stinging hairs on the leaf and stem, another identifying feature of the plant. The best time to pick nettle is in the spring when it is less than five inches tall. Later in the season, eating plants that have flowered can cause an upset stomach and irritate the kidneys.

104

PREPARATION: Nettles must be lightly steamed, boiled, or sautéed to neutralize the stinging hairs. It can be used as a substitute for spinach. The water the nettle was cooked in can be used for tea or in soups. Nettle can be dried and frozen for later use.

Nettles have been used to treat joint pain and muscle aches, and relieve season allergies. They are highly nutritious, and are a good source to meet the daily recommended requirements for calcium and iron.

NETTLES NUTRITION INFORMATION

Nettles are an excellent source of Vitamin A, and a good source of fiber

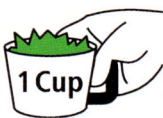

1 Cup

FIBER VITAMIN A

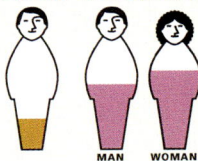

MAN WOMAN

HEART FRIENDLY
- Low in fat
- Very low in sodium

NUTRITION INFORMATION	
Per serving - 1 cup	
Energy	37 kcal
Protein	2 g
Carbohydrate	7 g
Fat	0.1 g
Calories from fat	2 %
Dietary Fiber	6 g
Cholesterol	NA
Sodium	4 mg
Vitamin A	1790 IU
Vitamin C	NA*
Iron	1 mg
	*Not Available

High Bush Salmonberry
Salmonberry

NATIVE NAMES: Was'x'aan tléigu *(Tlingit)*, Alagnan *(Unangam Tunuu)*

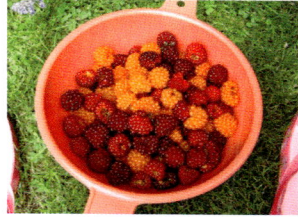

In Alaska the salmonberry ranges from Southcentral Alaska to the Kenai Peninsula and Southeast Alaska. They are mainly found in moist woods, at the base of mountains, or along roadsides. These berries may be red or orange when ripe and are ready for harvesting in mid to late summer depending on the location. The fruit has a sweet tart flavor and is related to the raspberry. There is a similar berry called salmonberry in Western and Southwestern Alaska, with a very different taste.

PREPARATION: Fresh salmonberry shoots, flowers and leaves and berries are edible. Salmonberry shoots can be eaten raw, or added to dishes and stir fried. The flowers can be added to salads, or used to make teas, and the berries are great for jams, pies, syrups, Eskimo ice cream, or just eaten by themselves.

CAUTION: Salmonberry flowers should be used fresh or completely dried. When partially dried they can be mildly toxic.

The most common theory about how salmonberries got their name is based on their resemblance to the color of salmon eggs, but one Chinook legend tells how Coyote had to put salmonberries in the mouth of each salmon he caught in order to have continued luck with fishing.

105

SALMONBERRY NUTRITION INFORMATION

Salmonberries are an excellent source of Vitamin A, and a good source of Vitamin C and iron

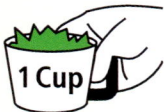

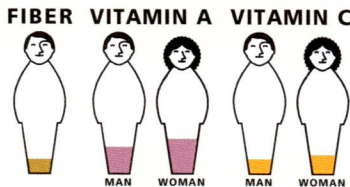

1 Cup

FIBER   VITAMIN A   VITAMIN C

MAN   WOMAN   MAN   WOMAN

HEART FRIENDLY
- Low in fat
- Very low in sodium

NUTRITION INFORMATION	
Per serving - 1 cup: raw	
Calories	68
Protein	1 g
Carbohydrate	15 g
Fat	0
Calories from fat	0 %
Saturated fat	NT*
Dietary Fiber	3 g
Cholesterol	NT*
Sodium	20 mg
Vitamin A	719 IU
Vitamin C	13 mg
Iron	1 mg

*Not Tested

Seaweed

Kelp, Black, Ribbon

NATIVE NAMES: **Elquaq** *(Yup'ik)*,
Laak'ásk *(Tlingit)*,
Qahngux̂ - *Seaweed, kelp in general*
(Unangam Tunuu)

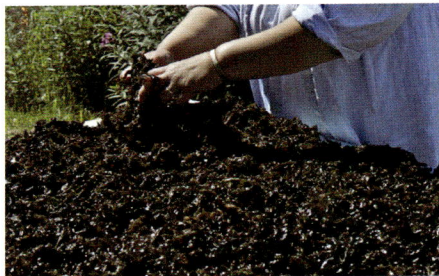

Seaweed is available along
the Southeast Alaska coast,

ANTHC

Gulf of Alaska, and Aleutian Islands. Green in color, it turns
black when dried. It has three growth seasons: winter, spring
and summer, but it's best to harvest in the early spring (April
and May). Harvest times vary each year in relation to changes in
temperature, sun, and rain. The seaweed should be 8 to 15 inches
long, elastic and stretchy when it is ready to be harvested.

PREPARATION: Seaweed can be eaten raw, dried, or boiled.
It makes a good snack eaten like "popcorn." It keeps indefinitely
if dried thoroughly, and is best dried in the sun. It may be added
to salads, fish stews, and soups for flavor.

*Seaweed is a prized food to the Tlingit, Haida, and Tsimshian.
Dried seaweed tastes different from one Southeast community
to another as each has a distinct taste. Recipes are shared from
generation to generation. Traditionally, fresh or dried seaweed was
used as a natural laxative, and to draw out infections. The salt and
iodine in seaweed is used to soothe a sore throat.*

106

SEAWEED NUTRITION INFORMATION

*Nutrient data based on
black seaweed

Seaweed is an excellent
source of Vitamin A, and a
good source of fiber

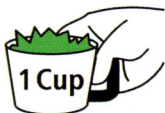

FIBER **VITAMIN A**

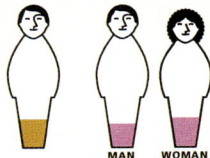

MAN   WOMAN

1 Cup

HEART FRIENDLY
• Fat free

NUTRITION INFORMATION	
Per serving - 1 cup: dried	
Calories	40
Protein	4 g
Carbohydrate	6 g
Fat	0
Calories from fat	0 %
Saturated fat	0
Dietary Fiber	5 g
Cholesterol	NT*
Sodium	145 mg
Vitamin A	613 IU
Vitamin C	2 mg
Iron	1 mg

*Not Tested

Sea Lovage
Beach Lovage

NATIVE NAMES: Tukaayuq *(Yup'ik),*
Tukkaayuk *(Tlingit)*

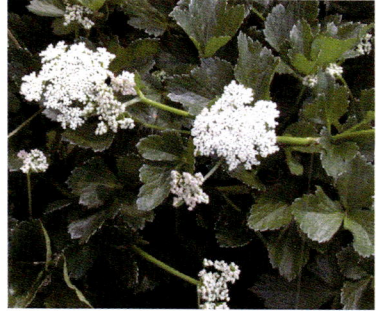

Alaska Plant Materials Center

Sea lovage is a member of the parsley family and grows in sandy and gravelly areas along the coast. It can grow up to two feet high and has three shiny leaflets, with white or pink colored flowers. Sea lovage is sweet, mild, and tender. For the best texture and flavor, it is picked before other leaves and grasses grow around it when the leaves are half-grown. Sea lovage is known as "petrúshki" in the Kodiak Island area.

PREPARATION: The Iñupiaq eat the leaves raw in seal oil. Fresh sea lovage has a pungent spicy flavor. When stored in oil, it is milder and sweeter. Sea lovage can be used as a seasoning in dishes: boiled or baked with fish; added to soups and stews; or used as a substitute for celery or parsley in recipes.

107

Sea lovage is used as a seasoning for fish dishes or salads in the Aleutians. Wild green lovers use sea lovage much like spinach or swiss chard.

NO NUTRITION INFORMATION AVAILABLE

Sourdock
Arctic Dock, Sorrel

NATIVE NAMES:
Quaqciq *(Yup'ik)*,
Qunnarliiq *(Alutiiq)*,
Quagaq *(Iñupiaq)*,
Aluungix̂ *(Unangam Tunuu -
Atka dialect)*, Tl'aak̲'wách' *(Tlingit)*

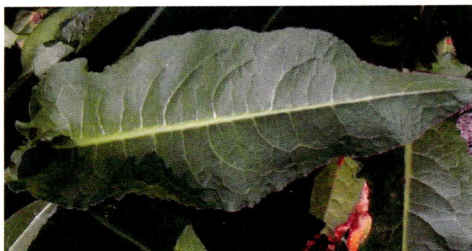

Alaska Plant Materials Center

Sourdock grows in wet places along lakes and rivers. It can be picked all summer and fall as soon as the leaves are big enough. It can be harvested in the winter if the plant grows near a spring which helps prevent the ground from freezing. Sourdock leaves and stems are edible. The large plant leaves have a sour taste.

PREPARATION: Traditionally in the North, large quantities of sourdock are cooked and then stored to ferment with seal fat and berries, to eat in the winter. The acidic qualities of sourdock have been used to pickle and preserve foods, including trout, for the long winter. Stems can be made into jam.

"My favorite wild plant is sourdock. I have fond memories of picking sourdock with my grandmother. She filled an old flour or sugar sack, put it in a huge pot, added sugar, and boiled it with lots of water. The juice was put in a big stainless steel pot and that would be our juice when we were at camp. It had a unique flavor and almost tasted like guava juice."

– Emily Hughes, Teller

SOURDOCK NUTRITION INFORMATION

Sourdock is an excellent source of Vitamin A & C

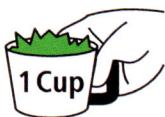

VITAMIN A   **VITAMIN C**

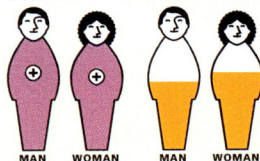

MAN   WOMAN   MAN   WOMAN

1 Cup

HEART FRIENDLY
- Low in fat
- Low calorie

NUTRITION INFORMATION	
Per serving - 1 cup: young leaves	
Calories	34
Protein	2 g
Carbohydrate	5 g
Fat	1 g
Calories from fat	14 %
Saturated fat	NT*
Dietary Fiber	NT*
Cholesterol	NT*
Sodium	NT*
Vitamin A	9520 IU
Vitamin C	54 mg
Iron	1 mg

*Not Tested

Tundra Tea
*Hudson Bay Tea,
Labrador Tea,
Eskimo Tea*

NATIVE NAMES: Ayuq *(Yup'ik)*,
Kenunghdza *(Dena'ina)*,
Caa'uq *(Alutiiq)*,
S'ikshaldéen *(Tlingit)*, Tilaaqiuq *(Iñupiaq)*

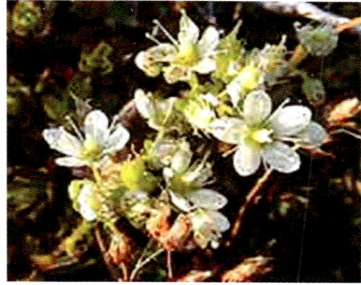
Alaska Plant Materials Center

Tundra tea is a shrub with distinct leaves, a brownish underside
and flowers that are white or pink. It grows throughout Alaska,
except on the Aleutian Islands. It is commonly found in the
tundra, bog, and spruce forest environments. It is a very popular
traditional beverage with medicinal properties that are considered
safe when used in moderation.

**CAUTION: Consuming large quantities can have
toxic effects.**

PREPARATION: Tundra tea is made by pouring boiling
water over the leaves and steeping gently. The leaves can also be
used as a spice to flavor other teas, sauces, meats and stews. It is
said the older, darker leaves "make the tastiest tea."

*The Yup'ik use tundra tea to soothe an upset stomach. The
Dena'ina also use the tea for heartburn, colds, and arthritis, as a
wash for sores, and a laxative.*

**TUNDRA TEA
NUTRITION INFORMATION**

1 OZ

HEART FRIENDLY
- Fat free
- Low calorie

NUTRITION INFORMATION	
Per serving - 1 oz tea	
Calories	2
Protein	0
Carbohydrate	0
Fat	0
Calories from fat	0 %
Saturated fat	0
Dietary Fiber	NT*
Cholesterol	0
Sodium	313 mg
Vitamin A	0
Vitamin C	1 mg
Iron	0

*Not Tested

Wild Celery

Indian Celery, Cow Parsnip

NATIVE NAMES: Ikiituk *(Yup'ik)*,
Vgyuun *(Alutiiq)*, Yaana.eit *(Tlingit)*,
Ikuusuk *(Iñupiaq)*,
Saaqudax̂ *(Unangam Tunuu)*

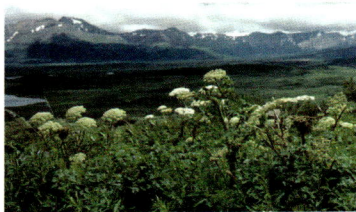

U.S. Fish & Wildlife Service

Wild celery is an important Alaska Native medicine and food plant. It grows up to eight feet tall, bears small white flowers, and has a strong smell. It grows along the coast where it is moist and among the beach grasses.

CAUTION: Great care should be taken to identify wild celery correctly, because there are plants in the same family with similar-looking flowers that are deadly poisonous, such as water hemlock.

110

PREPARATION: The stems of wild celery can be eaten raw or cooked. They should always be peeled before consuming. It is a great replacement for regular celery in many recipes, stews, casseroles, and stir fries. It has a similar but much stronger taste than sea lovage.

The dried stem of the plant was used as a drinking straw by new mothers in earlier days.

WILD CELERY NUTRITION INFORMATION*

*Nutrient data based on domestic celery

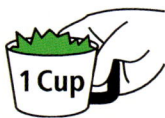

1 Cup

HEART FRIENDLY
- Low calorie
- Low in sodium

NUTRITION INFORMATION	
Per serving - 1 cup: cooked	
Calories	14
Protein	1 g
Carbohydrate	3 g
Fat	0
Calories from fat	0 %
Saturated fat	0
Dietary Fiber	1 g
Cholesterol	0
Sodium	68 mg
Vitamin A	87 IU
Vitamin C	5 mg
Iron	0

Wild Rhubarb
Alaskan Rhubarb

NATIVE NAMES: Angukaq *(Yup'ik),*
Tl'aak'wách' *(Tlingit),*
Quuguulnaadax̂ *(Unangam Tunuu - Nikolski dialect),* Qurjulliq *(Iñupiaq)*

Alaska Plant Materials Center

Wild rhubarb is a large herb that can grow to over six feet tall. It is common in Western and Interior Alaska. It grows in woods and along streams in the inland area.

PREPARATION: Wild rhubarb is often used for rhubarb in many pie and jam recipes. Traditionally, the stems and leaves were boiled and eaten plain. Other popular ways to eat wild rhubarb include eating the raw tips with peanut butter, or cutting the wild rhubarb into green salads.

"One food I still eat a lot of is cooked wild rhubarb mixed with blackberries. It has a lot of vitamins that are missing in our diet. It provides good nourishment. I learned from my mother, mother-in-law and other elders about the greens that are edible and most importantly, when to pick them. Wild rhubarb grows along the bank of the lake where we have our summer camp. You have to pick them while they are young and tender."

– Mary Schaeffer, Kotzebue

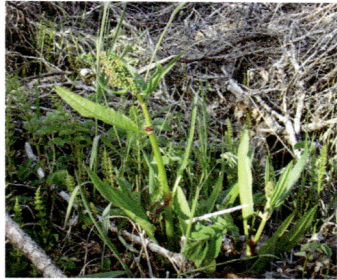

111

WILD RHUBARB NUTRITION INFORMATION

Wild rhubarb is an excellent source of Vitamins A & C

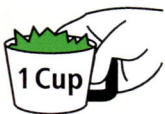

VITAMIN A   VITAMIN C

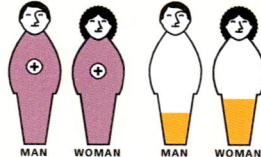

MAN   WOMAN   MAN   WOMAN

1 Cup

HEART FRIENDLY
• Fat free

NUTRITION INFORMATION	
Per serving - 1 cup: leaves	
Calories	49
Protein	3 g
Carbohydrate	8 g
Fat	0
Calories from fat	0 %
Saturated fat	NT*
Dietary Fiber	NT*
Cholesterol	NT*
Sodium	NT*
Vitamin A	3584 IU
Vitamin C	26 mg
Iron	NT*

*Not Tested

Wild Rice

Chocolate Lily, Indian Rice, Kamchatka Lily, Riceroot

NATIVE NAMES:
Paraluruat *(Yup'ik),*
Laaqaq *(Aleut),* **Koox** *(Tlingit)*

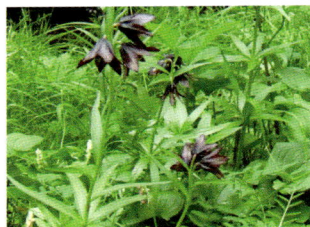

Robert Gorman

Wild rice is found along the coast, stream banks, and marshy areas of Southcentral and Southeast Alaska, as well as the Aleutian Chain. It has a green stem and flowers that are dark purple or nearly black in color. Wild rice can grow 1 to 2 feet tall. It is harvested summer through fall. Wild rice has an aroma that is unforgettable.

PREPARATION: The bulb of the plant is the source of the rice. People usually dig with their hands to obtain the bulb. The Dena'ina use the bulb for food by breaking it apart and soaking it overnight to remove any bitter taste. They then boil it about 1 hour and then pour off the water. It is mixed with any kind of oil before eating. Wild rice can also be eaten raw or dried, and is used in casseroles, soups, and stews, or as a side dish.

– Tananaina Plant Lore

112

WILD RICE NUTRITION INFORMATION*

*Nutrient data based on chocolate lilly bulbs

Wild rice is a good source of fiber

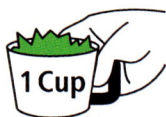

FIBER

1 Cup

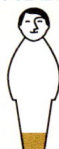

HEART FRIENDLY
● Low in fat
● Very low in sodium

NUTRITION INFORMATION	
Per serving - 1 cup	
Calories	166
Protein	7 g
Carbohydrate	35 g
Fat	1 g
Calories from fat	3 %
Saturated fat	0
Dietary Fiber	3 g
Cholesterol	0
Sodium	5 mg
Vitamin A	5 IU
Vitamin C	0
Iron	1 mg

Willow Leaves

NATIVE NAMES: Enrilnguaq *(Yup'ik)*,
Ch'áal' *(Tlingit)*, Akutuqpalik *(Iñupiaq)*

There are many different types of
willow in Alaska. Some willow are bitter
and regarded as inedible, but all are
safe to eat. One favorite to eat is Surah,
which has a refeshing aftertaste. Look
for leaves that are long and narrow,
smooth on both sides, with smooth
margins and a darker shade of green
above. The bark of many willows is
bitter tasting due to the natural aspirin
it contains. Herbalists find willow bark
teas, tinctures and salves to be effective
and lack the side effects of the synthetic drug. The willow is a
favorite food of moose.

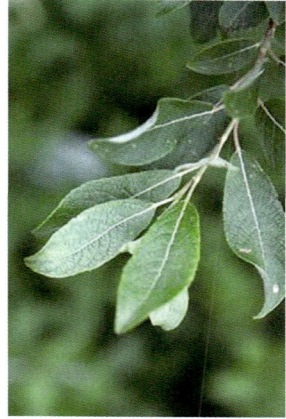

Alaska Plant Materials Center

PREPARATION: Pick willow leaves in early spring when
bright green and 1/2 - 1 1/2 inch long. Nibble leaves as a snack, or
add to salads, sandwiches, or casseroles.

*"In the spring, the wild willow leaves start sprouting.
That is one of the best times to pick the leaves.
After picking, we soak them in seal oil in jars for use
as a side dish in the summer."*
                                               – Emily Hughes, Teller

WILLOW LEAF NUTRITION INFORMATION

Willow leaf is an
excellent source of
Vitamins A & C

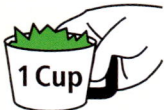

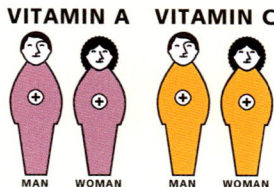

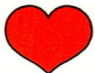

1 Cup

VITAMIN A

MAN   WOMAN

VITAMIN C

MAN   WOMAN

HEART FRIENDLY
- Low in fat

NUTRITION INFORMATION	
Per serv. - 1 cup: young leaves, chopped	
Calories	67
Protein	3 g
Carbohydrate	11 g
Fat	1 g
Calories from fat	12 %
Saturated fat	NT*
Dietary Fiber	NT*
Cholesterol	NT*
Sodium	NT*
Vitamin A	10285 IU
Vitamin C	105 mg
Iron	1 mg

*Not Tested

Stinkweed

Wormwood, Caribou Leaves, Alaskan Sage

NATIVE NAMES:
Caiggluk *(Yup'ik),* Charighik *(Iñupiaq)*

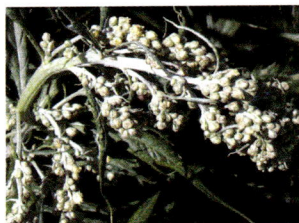

Alaska Plant Materials Center

Stinkweed can be found in northern communities along the Arctic Ocean and Bering Sea, and southward along Southeast's Northern Panhandle. It can grow 1 to 3 feet tall, has narrow leaves yellow-green to brown in color, with a silvery underside and ball shaped flowers. Stinkweed has a distinct minty smell, hence the name "stinkweed." It has both medicinal and food use: the leaves are harvested before the plant flowers for use as a spice, with leaves and flowers harvested for medicinal use.

CAUTION: Consuming large quantities can affect the central nervous system causing convulsions, and comas. The plant should be avoided by pregnant or breast-feeding women.

114

PREPARATION: Stinkweed is very bitter. Its leaves can be dried and used as a spice. Leaves and flowers can be finely chopped and boiled until dark for a medicinal tea. Other traditional methods include wetting the stinkweed and applying directly to sores and cuts. It can also be wrapped around a hot pad to treat an earache.

Alaska Native people have long known the medicinal qualities of stinkweed. Stinkweed teas are used to fight infection from colds, the flu, a sore throat, and upset stomachs. It is also applied externally as a treatment for body aches, cuts, rashes, and sores. Bristol Bay residents tie stinkweed into bundles and slap against the body during steam baths to relieve pain.

Stinkweed is not regarded as a food. However its popularity with Alaska Native people as a traditional medicinal plant is the reason it is included in this guide.

NO NUTRITION INFORMATION AVAILABLE

"We always have tundra tea, and mix it with a little bit of store-bought tea. Everyone always wants to have tundra tea at potlatches."

– Audrey Armstrong, Huslia

"There were greens that we picked along the slough or river. We would blanch the gathered greens and eat them with seal oil. One of the greens, sourdock, we would blanch, drain the water, and place in a barrel. Later adding crowberries and mix them together for winter use. We'd eat it as is or add to akutaq."

– Jeannette Smith, Wasilla (originally from Hooper Bay)

I love to go berry picking with my mom. It gives us much satisfaction to bring home full buckets to our families. My mom taught me how to make delicious desserts with berries, but my favorite recipe is the

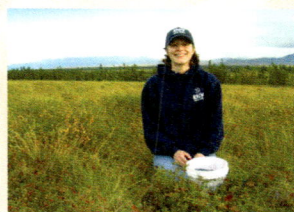

"Dr. Nagaruk is a cancer survivor who desperately missed her Native foods (especially berries) while she was in Seattle, WA for cancer treatment.

easiest: Pour frozen berries into a bowl. Eat with spoon. Canned milk, sprinkle of sugar optional. Mmmmmmmm. I think I'll go eat a bowl of berries!"

– Nora Nagaruk, MD Nome (originally from Unalakleet)

Other Foods

Sailor Boy Pilot Bread

Pilot Boy Crackers

NATIVE NAMES: Suggaliq *(Yup'ik)*, Qaqqulaaq *(Iñupiaq)*

According to Tlingit elders, Pilot Bread was introduced along with sugar and rice with the arrival of the first white men by ship. It continues to be a staple for many families today.

Karen Morgan

PREPARATION: Serves as a hand-held base for many foods, keeps a long time, and travels well. Pilot bread, dried fish, and tea are common foods to take hunting and fishing.

Alaskans may not live by Pilot Bread alone, but they profess an unmatched devotion to the round, durable, unsalted crackers that are the staff of life for villagers, cabin-dwellers and a few city-folk. One elder would eat Pilot Bread every day if he could, "I like that whipped cheese on it, but I have to drive 34 miles to buy it, so I don't always have it." Another likes "eating it in soup, like moose soup or something."

– Anchorage Daily News, November 6, 2007

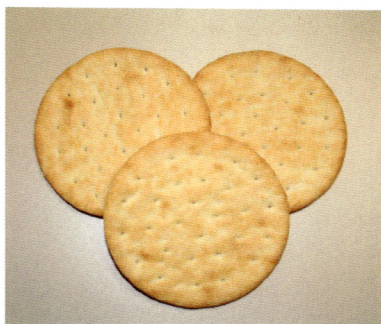

117

PILOT BREAD NUTRITION INFORMATION

NUTRITION INFORMATION	
Per serving - 25 g: 1 piece	
Calories	100
Protein	2 g
Carbohydrate	18 g
Fat	3 g
Calories from fat	20 %
Saturated fat	0
Dietary Fiber	1 g
Cholesterol	0 g
Sodium	130 mg
Vitamin A	0 IU
Vitamin C	0 g
Iron	1 mg

Eskimo Ice Cream

NATIVE NAMES: Akutaq *(Yup'ik)*,
Akutuq *(Iñupiaq)*

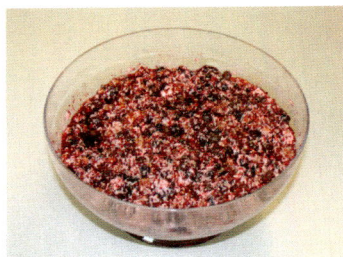

Patricia Bunyan

Eskimo ice cream, or akutaq, is made for special occasions: celebrations, funerals, when a boy gets his first animal, and holidays. Akutaq (pronounced A-GOO-DUK) is Yu'pik and means "blended one" or "mix them together." Recipes differ from one Alaska region to another, and it is typically made with Crisco, berries, ground fish, or seal oil.

PREPARATION: Berries, fish, or meat can be used as ingredients to make Eskimo ice cream a dessert or a meal. Eskimo ice cream is an excellent trail food since it packs easily and can be eaten frozen.

118

Eskimo ice cream is a well-known Alaska Native favorite. In times past hunters would bring "akutaq" along with them on hunting trips as a survival food.

ESKIMO ICE CREAM NUTRITION INFORMATION

* Detailed nutrients of the five usual ingredients: a hard fat like back fat, a soft fat like seal oil or vegetable oil, liquid like water or juice, sweetening, and other foods like berries, fish, or greens.

NUTRITION INFORMATION	
Per serving - 1/2 cup: Salmonberry Agutak	
Calories	331
Protein	1 g
Carbohydrate	16 g
Fat	30 g
Calories from fat	82 %
Saturated fat	7 g SFA
Dietary Fiber	1 g
Cholesterol	0
Sodium	30 mg
Vitamin A	23 RE
Vitamin C	1 mg
Iron	1 mg

Akutaq (Eskimo Ice Cream)

Akutaq is a Yup'ik word that means "mix them together," but white men called it "Eskimo Ice Cream." Akutaq is made in many different ways. This recipe was made by Natives a long, long time ago for survival. When Natives went out to go hunting, they brought along akutaq. Akutaq can also be made with moose meat and fat, caribou meat and fat, fish, seal oil, berries.

This was a healthy and tasty treat for Alaska Natives a long time ago; they never used sugar. Each family makes akutaq a little differently. This is how my family makes our akutaq. There aren't any real instructions on how to make this recipe because we make it the way we were taught and we pass it down to our kids that way.

The traditional way to make akutaq is to let them watch and learn. And when we are done making it, we draw a shape of a cross in the middle of the akutaq with our finger. Then we take each type of berry from the akutaq (unless there is only one type of berry) and a pinch of the mixture and throw it into the fire. When I do that, I have to say, "Tamarpeci nerluci." In English it means "All of you eat!"

– www.ankn.uaf.edu

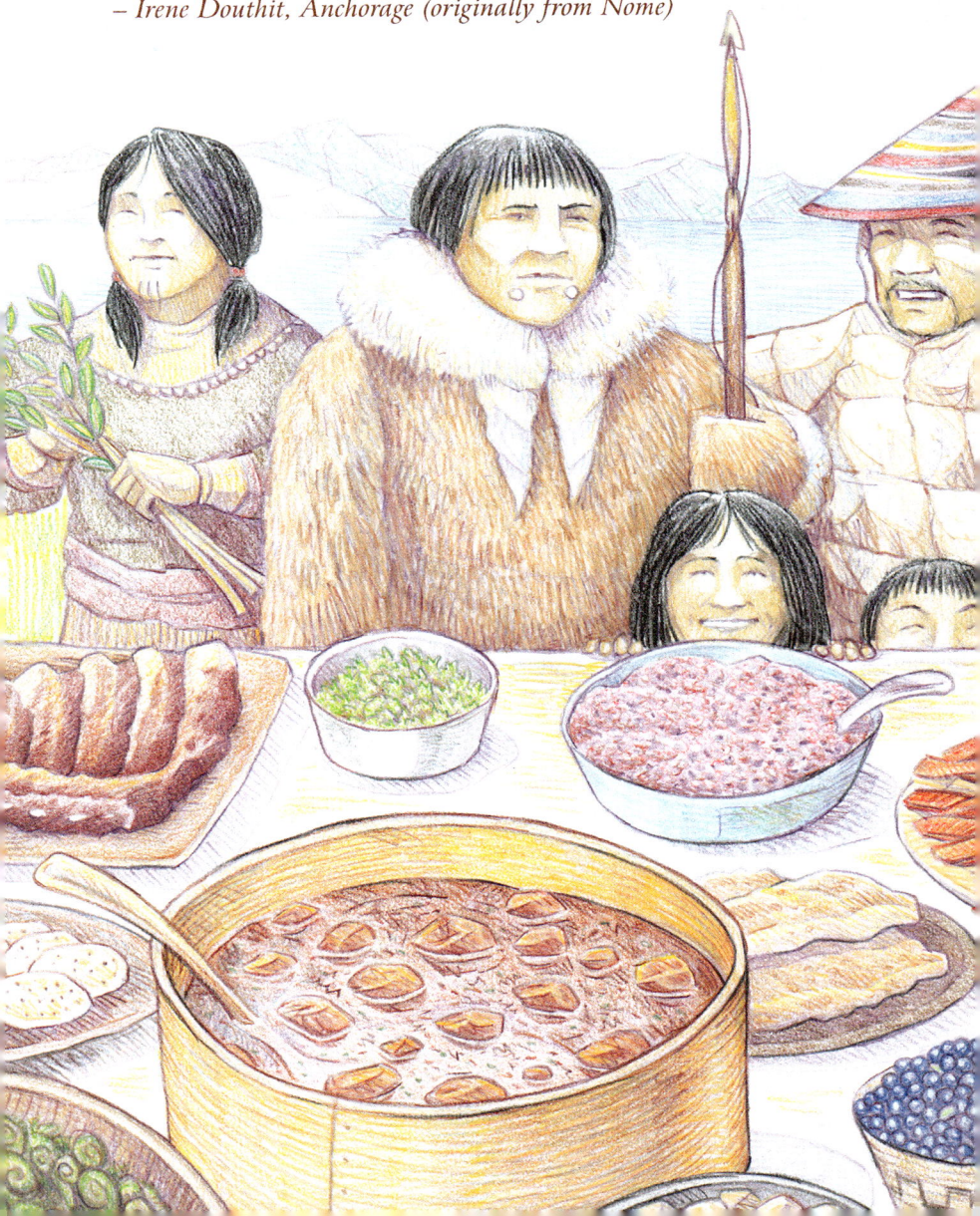

"Native food tastes better when it is eaten with a big group of friends and family . . . when we put all our Native foods together, it is a feast."

– Irene Douthit, Anchorage (originally from Nome)

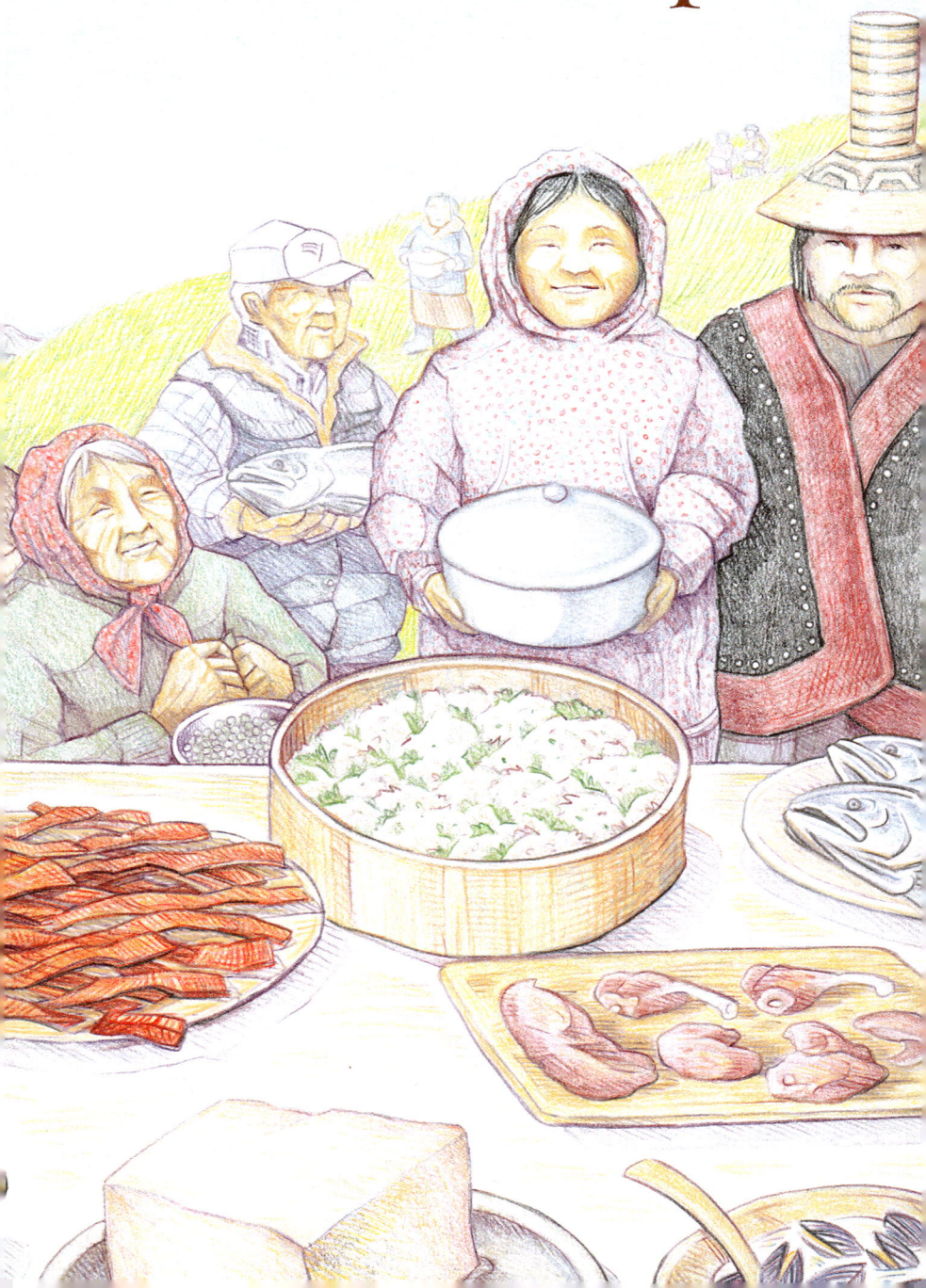

Recipes

RECIPE TABLE OF CONTENTS

Fish rack at Kotlik   *ANTHC - Division of Environmental Health & Engineering*

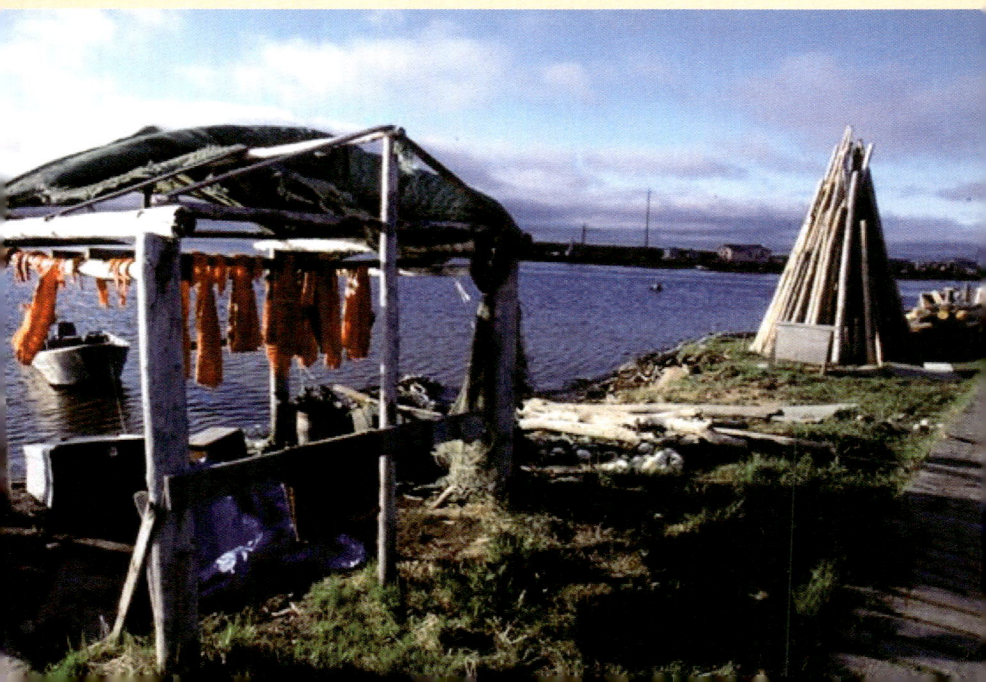

Arctic Fajitas

INGREDIENTS:

1 to 2 lb moose, caribou, reindeer,
   or musk ox meat

1 green pepper

1 medium onion

Soy sauce to taste

1 medium tomato

Sour cream or yogurt for topping

Salt and pepper to taste

2-3 cloves crushed garlic

Additional spices as desired

Fresh flour tortillas or whole wheat flour tortillas

NUTRITION INFORMATION	
Makes 8 fajitas. Per fajita:	
Calories	306
Protein	25.1 g
Carbohydrate	29.4 g
Fat	9.6 g
Saturated fat	2.7 g
Dietary Fiber	0.8 g
Cholesterol	76.6 mg
Sodium	557 mg
Vitamin A	260.4 IU
Vitamin C	19.9 mg
Iron	5.3 mg

INSTRUCTIONS: Slice meat in the thinnest strips possible
(partially frozen meat makes this easier). Fry meat in oil in
skillet till brown, Add salt, pepper, garlic, and a dash of soy
sauce. Add peppers and cook until peppers are half cooked. Put
your hot filling in a fresh tortilla; add fresh tomatoes, onions and
sour cream.

*– From "Build Strong Families - Arctic Home Cooking", 2nd Edition,
by Maniilaq Association Employees, Kotzebue, Alaska*

124

Moose Meat, Gravy and Rice

INGREDIENTS:

1 lb moose meat

1 teaspoon garlic powder

Salt to taste

Pepper to taste

3 to 4 cups water

¼ cup soy sauce

1 bunch broccoli

½ bunch cauliflower

1 small can mushrooms

4 tablespoons cornstarch (or flour)

½ cup water

NUTRITION INFORMATION	
Serves 4. Per serving:	
Calories	357
Protein	35.5 g
Carbohydrate	50.8 g
Fat	2.7 g
Saturated fat	0.4 g
Dietary Fiber	7.1 g
Cholesterol	61.3 mg
Sodium	1082.5 mg
Vitamin A	956.3 IU
Vitamin C	173.6 mg
Iron	7.2 mg

125

INSTRUCTIONS: Cut meat into bite size pieces and brown in a large fry pan. Add salt, pepper and garlic powder. When meat is well done and brown, add water and soy sauce; bring to a boil, then let simmer 45 minutes to one hour. Cut vegetables into bite size pieces and add to meat. Let simmer for 15 minutes. Mix cornstarch into ½ cup water. Mix very well and add to meat, and vegetables, stirring constantly until desired thickness. Cook for about 5 minutes or until gravy is done. Serve over steamed rice.

– From "Build Strong Families - Arctic Home Cooking", 2nd Edition,
by Maniilaq Association Employees, Kotzebue, Alaska

Caribou Soup

INGREDIENTS:

1 gallon plastic storage bag of caribou

3-4 tablespoons cooking oil

Chopped onions to taste

Chopped carrots

Chopped celery

1 cup rice

1 cup macaroni/noodles

1 tablespoon parsley

Garlic salt, to taste

Onion salt to taste

1 tablespoon curry (optional)

1 large pot of water

Salt and pepper to taste

NUTRITION INFORMATION	
Per 1 cup serving:	
Calories	98.4
Protein	9.1 g
Carbohydrate	11.5 g
Fat	1.7 g
Saturated fat	0.02 g
Dietary Fiber	0.24 g
Cholesterol	
Sodium	173.3 mg
Vitamin A	3856.8 IU
Vitamin C	3.6 mg
Iron	0.5 mg

INSTRUCTIONS: Cut the caribou meat into bite size pieces. Can use ribs, backbones or any pieces of meat with bones. Sauté in pot with cooking oil. Sprinkle a little bit of meat tenderizer if needed. Add salt, garlic salt, onion salt, and parsley flakes. Pepper is optional. Add onion, celery, and carrots, then sauté in oil with meat. Cook until meat is brown, about a half hour. Add about 2 ½ quarts water to cover meat and vegetables. Boil for one hour; stir to prevent sticking. Salt to taste. Add potatoes, rice, and macaroni; cook another half hour on low simmer.

– From "Build Strong Families - Arctic Home Cooking", 2nd Edition, by Maniilaq Association Employees, Kotzebue, Alaska

Caribou Stew

INGREDIENTS:

1 pound caribou meat

3 medium potatoes

1 onion (chopped)

1 package mixed vegetables

1 can of tomatoes

1 tablespoon beef soup seasoning base

1/2 teaspoon Tabasco pepper sauce

3 tablespoons Spike seasoning

Rice

NUTRITION INFORMATION	
Per serving - 2 cups:	
Calories	513
Protein	32 g
Carbohydrate	83 g
Fat	5 g
Calories from Fat	8 %
Saturated fat	2 g
Dietary Fiber	9 g
Cholesterol	82 mg
Sodium	1661 mg
Vitamin A	4500 IU
Vitamin C	37 mg
Iron	8 mg

INSTRUCTIONS: Boil caribou for 30 minutes. Add rest of ingredients and seasoning to taste. Simmer for 1 hour.

– *Jeannette M. Smith, Wasilla (originally from Hooper Bay)*

127

Quick Caribou Taco Soup

INGREDIENTS:

2 lbs. ground caribou

1 chopped onion

2 cans diced tomatoes and green chilis

2 cans whole kernel corn

2 cans ranch style beans

1 package taco seasoning

1 package ranch dressing mix

Grated cheese

NUTRITION INFORMATION	
Per serving - 1 1/2 cups:	
Calories	395
Protein	40 g
Carbohydrate	34 g
Fat	12 g
Calories from Fat	27 %
Saturated fat	5 g
Dietary Fiber	6 g
Cholesterol	128 mg
Sodium	834 mg
Vitamin A	900 IU
Vitamin C	16 mg
Iron	9.9 mg

INSTRUCTIONS: Brown ground meat with onion until the meat is brown and onion is clear. Drain the grease. Put in a large pot and add the rest of the ingredients. Simmer 15 - 20 minutes. Serve with oyster crackers or tortilla chips and grated cheese.

– *Jeannette M. Smith, Wasilla (originally from Hooper Bay)*

Grilled Caribou or Moose Marinade

INGREDIENTS:

Caribou or moose steaks

2/3 cup soy sauce

1/4 cup olive oil

6 garlic cloves (cut or minced)

2 teaspoons ground ginger

2 teaspoons dry mustard

2 tablespoons molasses

Bacon

INSTRUCTIONS: Mix soy sauce, oil, garlic, ginger, mustard, and molasses. Place thick bacon around the steak and hold in place with tooth picks. Brine for an hour or overnight then cook on a grill.

– *Jeannette M. Smith, Wasilla (originally from Hooper Bay)*

128

Baked Moose Bones

INGREDIENTS:

2 lbs. moose bones (or caribou bones)

3 small potatoes, peeled and diced

4 stalks celery

4 carrots

1 medium onion

INSTRUCTIONS: Put the bones in a roasting pan. Peel and dice the potatoes and carrots, and chop the celery and onion. Add the vegetables and some water to the pan. Bake moose bones for two hours at 400 ° F. Bake caribou bones at 375 ° F for one to two hours.

– *Natasha Nelson, Ekwok*

NUTRITION INFORMATION	
Per serving -3 oz:	
Calories	977
Protein	4 g
Carbohydrate	29 g
Fat	94 g
Calories from Fat	87 %
Saturated fat	31 g
Dietary Fiber	5 g
Cholesterol	50 mg
Sodium	81 mg
Vitamin A	10395 IU
Vitamin C	31 mg
Iron	1.9 mg

Beaver Pot Roast

INGREDIENTS:

Beaver

Flour

2 small onions

2 bay leaves

Salt and pepper

NUTRITION INFORMATION	
Serves 4. Per serving:	
Calories	218.8
Protein	28.7 g
Carbohydrate	11.5 g
Fat	5.6 g
Saturated fat	*
Dietary Fiber	1 g
Cholesterol	*
Sodium	59.5 mg
Vitamin A	10.75 IU
Vitamin C	5 mg
Iron	8.5 mg

INSTRUCTIONS: Cut small beaver hindquarters into pieces. Dip in flour and brown in a dutch oven. Add onions and bay leaves. Add salt and pepper to taste. Cover and let cook until fork tender.

– *From "Out of Alaska's Kitchens", 1961*

Baked Spring Squirrel or Muskrat

INGREDIENTS:

3-4 spring squirrels or muskrats, skinned and gutted

1/2 onion

Salt and pepper to taste

Garlic powder to taste

Butter

NUTRITION INFORMATION	
Serves 6. Per serving:	
Calories	302.5
Protein	31.7 g
Carbohydrate	1.5 g
Fat	18.1 g
Saturated fat	3.7 g
Dietary Fiber	0.3 g
Cholesterol	15.3 mg
Sodium	359.2 mg
Vitamin A	178.3 IU
Vitamin C	8.6 mg
Iron	10 mg

INSTRUCTIONS: Put the cleaned squirrel/muskrat in a baking pan lined with tin foil. Pat with butter, salt, pepper, and garlic to taste. Add onion chunks. Bake, uncovered, until browned and crispy at 350° F, for 30 minutes to an hour, depending on your stove. Serve with baked potatoes and/or carrots. The old timers ate them. They taste like springtime!

– *From "Out of Alaska's Kitchens", 1961*

Duck Soup

INGREDIENTS:

1-2 ducks, plucked, cleaned, and cut up

Fresh or dried onion

Salt and pepper to taste

1 handful of rice

1 handful or macaroni

NUTRITION INFORMATION	
Serves 6. Per serving:	
Calories	219.5
Protein	15.2 g
Carbohydrate	11.1 g
Fat	12.3 g
Saturated fat	4 g
Dietary Fiber	0.5 g
Cholesterol	63.7 mg
Sodium	239.3 mg
Vitamin A	71 IU
Vitamin C	5.2 mg
Iron	3.9 mg

INSTRUCTIONS: In a large pot, boil all parts, including feet, head, gizzard, heart, and liver. Boil 1/2 hour, then add 1 onion or dried onion to taste. Add uncooked rice and macaroni. Cook slowly until rice is cooked, about 45 minutes.

– *From "Out of Alaska's Kitchens", 1961*

Breast of Duck

130

INGREDIENTS:

Duck breasts

Salt and pepper

Flour

Butter

NUTRITION INFORMATION	
Serves 4. Per serving:	
Calories	204.8
Protein	15.7 g
Carbohydrate	8.2 g
Fat	12 g
Saturated fat	6.5 g
Dietary Fiber	04 g
Cholesterol	79.3 mg
Sodium	103 mg
Vitamin A	305.8 IU
Vitamin C	4.6 mg
Iron	3.9 mg

INSTRUCTIONS: Combine salt, pepper and flour and then coat breasts well in mixture. Arrange in shallow pan or roaster. Dot breasts with butter. Place in hot oven at 450° to 500° F. Cook 20 to 30 minutes, basting often. Reduce heat and cook longer, if well done meat is preferred.

– *From "Out of Alaska's Kitchens", 1961*

Baked Ptarmigan

INGREDIENTS:

3 lb ptarmigan

1/2 cup water

2 tablespoons vegetable oil

2 small potatoes

1 sliced onion, raw

1/2 cup carrots, raw

NUTRITION INFORMATION	
Serves 4. Per serving:	
Calories	285.8
Protein	30.5 g
Carbohydrate	17.7 g
Fat	9.4 g
Saturated fat	0.5 g*
Dietary Fiber	3.1 g
Cholesterol	22.9 mg
Sodium	308 mg*
Vitamin A	3160.9 IU
Vitamin C	19.9 mg
Iron	7.5 mg

INSTRUCTIONS: Place cleaned ptarmigan in a deep baking dish with a cover. Add a little bit of oil and water. Arrange freshly cut vegetables, like potatoes, onion, carrots, or your favorite vegetables, around the sides of the dish. Season to taste. Bake until tender.

– From "Out of Alaska's Kitchens", 1961

131

Seagull Egg Pie

INGREDIENTS:

2 seagull eggs

1 teaspoon vanilla

2 1/2 cups milk

1/2 cup sugar

Dash of salt

Nutmeg

Unbaked pie shell

NUTRITION INFORMATION	
Serves 8. Per serving:	
Calories	302
Protein	23.5 g
Carbohydrate	2.7 g
Fat	22.3 g
Saturated fat	7.6 g
Dietary Fiber	0.5 g
Cholesterol	92.3 mg
Sodium	407 mg
Vitamin A	781.5 IU
Vitamin C	1.2 mg
Iron	1.1 mg

INSTRUCTIONS: Beat eggs, sugar, salt, vanilla together. Add milk and beat for 5 minutes. Place in unbaked pie shell and sprinkle with nutmeg, before putting in oven. Bake for 45 minutes at 400° F.

– From "Out of Alaska's Kitchens", 1961

Fish Head Soup

INGREDIENTS:

2 medium king salmon heads (with lower
   jaws, gills and teeth removed and cut into
   quarters)

2 king salmon collars (tips)

2 tail end pieces

½ stick of butter

2 large onions (quartered)

4 stalks celery cut in 3-inch pieces

4 carrots peeled and cut in 3-inch pieces

4 potatoes (quartered)

6 chicken bouillon cubes

4 cups quart water

1 tablespoon dried parsley

NUTRITION INFORMATION	
Per serving - 2 cups:	
Calories	386
Protein	38 g
Carbohydrate	24 g
Fat	14 g
Calories from Fat	31 %
Saturated fat	7 g
Dietary Fiber	4 g
Cholesterol	94 mg
Sodium	1390 mg
Vitamin A	5550 IU
Vitamin C	28 mg
Iron	1.4 mg

132

INSTRUCTIONS: In large 3-gallon pot, boil onions, celery,
carrots, potatoes and bouillon cubes for 15 minutes. Place fish
over vegetables, sprinkle with parsley and steam with cover on for
20 minutes. Salt and pepper to taste. Serve with buttered Sailor
Boy crackers and tea.

– William Johnson

From June 1998 issue of Fishhead Soup,
a newsletter published by the Peer Outreach Project, Dillingham, AK

Sheefish Chowder

INGREDIENTS:

Sheefish

Salt to taste

1 onion

Flour

Carrots, if desired

NUTRITION INFORMATION	
Serves 5. Per serving:	
Calories	127.8
Protein	20.8 g
Carbohydrate	5.2 g
Fat	2.7 g
Saturated fat	0.4 g
Dietary Fiber	0.8 g
Cholesterol	50.8 mg
Sodium	289.2 mg
Vitamin A	2139.4 IU
Vitamin C	2 mg
Iron	0.7 mg

INSTRUCTIONS: Skin and clean fish while frozen. Boil with salt and remove bones. Flake it, add salt and onions. Thicken with flour. Add carrots if desired.

– *From "Out of Alaska's Kitchens", 1961*

Herring Egg Salad

INGREDIENTS:

1-2 cups herring eggs

Lettuce or baby greens, washed and dried

¼ cup carrots, grated

1 ½ green onions, finely sliced

¼ cup radishes, thinly sliced

1-2 tomatoes, diced

NUTRITION INFORMATION	
Per serving - 3/4 cup:	
Calories	38
Protein	5 g
Carbohydrate	5 g
Fat	1 g
Calories from Fat	25 %
Saturated fat	0
Dietary Fiber	1 g
Cholesterol	20 mg
Sodium	41 mg
Vitamin A	1379 IU
Vitamin C	6 mg
Iron	2 mg

INSTRUCTIONS: Mix lettuce or baby greens, carrots, green onions, radishes, and tomatoes together well. Add one to two cups of cooked, cooled herring eggs. Make sure the herring eggs are nice sized portions, rather then clumps of eggs. You can add light canola mayonnaise or a salad dressing of your choice.

– *Eleanor Batchelder, Anchorage (originally from Juneau)*

Baked Whitefish

INGREDIENTS:

1 medium sized whitefish

1 medium onion

Salt and pepper

1 ½ cups rice

3 ½ cups water

NUTRITION INFORMATION	
Serves 6. Per serving:	
Calories	331.8
Protein	24.9 g
Carbohydrate	40.5 g
Fat	7.2 g
Saturated fat	1.6 g
Dietary Fiber	1.1 g
Cholesterol	62.3 mg
Sodium	252.8 mg
Vitamin A	612.8 IU
Vitamin C	1.4 mg
Iron	2.5 mg

INSTRUCTIONS: Clean and scale fish. Lay fish down. Put onion inside fish. Add rice and water with fish. Bake at 350° F for 40 minutes. Do not overbake.

– *From "The Alaskan Grub Box" by Sis Laraux*

Boiled Fish

INGREDIENTS:

Whitefish, or other small fish

Salt

½ cup onion

NUTRITION INFORMATION	
Serves 4. Per serving:	
Calories	154
Protein	21.6 g
Carbohydrate	1.3 g
Fat	6.9 g
Saturated fat	1.6 g
Dietary Fiber	0.3 g
Cholesterol	62.3 mg
Sodium	349 mg
Vitamin A	611.8 IU
Vitamin C	1.1 mg
Iron	0.4 mg

INSTRUCTIONS: Scale and clean fish. Cut up and put in a kettle of water with salt and boil until done. Drain and serve with raw onions.

– *From "Out of Alaska's Kitchens", 1961*

King Salmon Roast

INGREDIENTS:

Salt and pepper

1 teaspoon dry mustard

1/2 cup sliced onion

3 tablespoons melted butter or olive oil

INSTRUCTIONS: Remove the scales from
the salmon and cut a piece suited to your
family. Wash fish in clear, cold water with a
teaspoon of table salt added. Wipe dry on a
paper towel. Place salmon in a small roaster, or
an oblong bread pan with 1 1/2 cups cold water; salt and pepper
and 1 teaspoon of dry mustard sprinkled over the fish, plus 1/2
cup sliced onion and 3 tablespoons of melted butter or oil. Roast
in oven 1 1/2 hours or until done.

– From "Out of Alaska's Kitchens", 1961

NUTRITION INFORMATION	
Per serving - 3 oz:	
Calories	156
Protein	17 g
Carbohydrate	1 g
Fat	10 g
Calories from Fat	56 %
Saturated fat	4 g
Dietary Fiber	0
Cholesterol	49 mg
Sodium	142 mg
Vitamin A	200 IU
Vitamin C	1 mg
Iron	1 mg

135

Salmon Bake

INGREDIENTS:

1 to 2 fillet of salmon

1 to 3 tablespoons of mayonnaise or mustard

Spike seasoning to taste

Garlic seasoning to taste

Bacon and onions to taste

INSTRUCTIONS: Cover the salmon with
mayonnaise or mustard and seasonings. Add
bacon and onion as desired on top. Cook
covered at 350° with foil for about 20 mintues.
Remove foil and bake another 20 minutes.

– Jeannette M. Smith, Wasilla (originally from Hooper Bay)

NUTRITION INFORMATION	
Per serving - 3 oz:	
Calories	148
Protein	17 g
Carbohydrate	6 g
Fat	7 g
Calories from Fat	40 %
Saturated fat	1 g
Dietary Fiber	1 g
Cholesterol	38 mg
Sodium	146 mg
Vitamin A	100 IU
Vitamin C	4 mg
Iron	1 mg

Easy Fish Pie

INGREDIENTS:

¼ lb cabbage, shredded

1 large carrot, chopped

1 large onion, chopped

2 tablespoons shortening

2 tablespoons butter

Salt and pepper

1 lb salmon, skinned and boiled (easier to debone when cooked)

1 cup cooked rice

Pie crust

NUTRITION INFORMATION	
Serves 5. Per serving:	
Calories	306.6
Protein	28.8 g
Carbohydrate	18.1 g
Fat	18.2 g
Saturated fat	6 g*
Dietary Fiber	1.7 g
Cholesterol	63.8 mg
Sodium	352 mg*
Vitamin A	2670 IU
Vitamin C	12.2 mg
Iron	1.5 mg

INSTRUCTIONS: Combine cabbage, carrot, and onion; simmer all vegetables in shortening and butter until tender. Add salt and pepper. In a 9x13 inch pan, line the bottom of the pan with pie crust. Leave some dough for top. Preheat oven to 350°. Line pan with crust and place ½ the rice on the bottom crust, then ½ the cooked vegetables, then add salmon (next layer). Add the rest of the vegetables and the remainder of the rice and the top crust.

Halibut is also very good in fish pie, but do not overcook. Canned salmon can also be used. Mix the rice with the vegetables, spread on bottom crust, fill, then add top crust.

Bake 45 minutes.

– *From "The Alaskan Grub Box", by Sis Laraux*

Pallas Buttercups, Salmon and Rice

INGREDIENTS:

2 lbs Pallas Buttercups

2 fillets of salmon

4 oz. seal oil

2 cups long grain white rice

NUTRITION INFORMATION	
Serves 6. Per serving:	
Calories	491
Protein	36.3 g
Carbohydrate	26 g
Fat	28.1 g
Saturated fat	4.1 g
Dietary Fiber	*
Cholesterol	68.6 mg
Sodium	68.7 mg
Vitamin A	8448.9 IU
Vitamin C	55.6 mg
Iron	6 mg

INSTRUCTIONS: Boil fresh fish in water. Take 1/2 of broth from boiled fish and put into another pan. Boil buttercups in the broth. Eat with seal oil on top and serve with rice and fish.

– From "Out of Alaska's Kitchens", 1961

Humpy & Sea Lovage Soup

INGREDIENTS:

Couple of humpies

1 teaspoon salt

1/2 cup sea lovage

1 onion, chopped

INSTRUCTIONS: Cut the cleaned humpies into thirds, heads and all. Place in pot and cover with water. Add salt to taste. Boil for 15-20 minutes. Add the sea lovage. Serve the broth in cups and fish on a plate, with seal oil on the side. Yummy!

– Irene Douthit, Anchorage (originally from Nome)

Smoked Bidarkis - Urritaq

INGREDIENTS:

30 cleaned, cooked, and sliced bidarkis

2/3 cup vegetable oil or seal oil

1 teaspoon of liquid smoke seasoning (adding too much can be bitter)

1 clove of fresh garlic minced

¼ onion

4 to 5 tablespoons of soy sauce

A dash of garlic salt

NUTRITION INFORMATION	
Per serving - 4 oz:	
Calories	238
Protein	19 g
Carbohydrate	4 g
Fat	18 g
Calories from Fat	0 %
Saturated fat	2 g
Dietary Fiber	0 g
Cholesterol	11 mg
Sodium	1016 mg
Vitamin A	2610 IU
Vitamin C	1 mg
Iron	16.5 mg

INSTRUCTIONS: In a large bowl, add your clean, sliced bidarkis and pour the oil and seasonings over the bidarkis. Cover the bowl and shake to mix the yummy flavor all over the bidarkis. This recipe becomes more awesome if you wish to add sliced octopus, herring eggs, and seaweed. Enjoy with friends. Native food always tastes better with a group of friends and family.

– Donna Malchoff, Anchorage (originally from Port Graham)

138

Seal Meat Soup

INGREDIENTS:

Seal

1/2 chopped onion

Sea salt to taste

2 cups uncooked rice

NUTRITION INFORMATION	
Per serving - 2 cups:	
Calories	322
Protein	32 g
Carbohydrate	38 g
Fat	4 g
Calories from Fat	0 %
Saturated fat	1 g
Dietary Fiber	1 g
Cholesterol	90 mg
Sodium	182 mg
Vitamin A	1050 IU
Vitamin C	1 mg
Iron	21.6 mg

INSTRUCTIONS: Thaw out seal meat the day before, and once thawed cut into bite size pieces. Add meat and 1/4 teaspoon sea salt and boil for 45 minutes to one hour. As the meat is boiling scrape off the residue and discard throughout the boiling process. After 45 minutes to one hour, add the uncooked rice and boil for another 20 minutes. If you choose to add vegetables like chopped carrots, celery, or potatoes, decrease the amount of rice.

– Jeannette Smith, Wasilla (originally from Hooper Bay)

Seaweed Rice Balls

INGREDIENTS:

2 tablespoons honey

4 tablespoons soy sauce

2 tablespoons sesame oil

1/4 teaspoon ground ginger

8 cups cooked rice

1/3 cup seasame seeds

2 cups roasted black seaweed, crushed

NUTRITION INFORMATION	
Per serving - 1/2 cup:	
Calories	42
Protein	3 g
Carbohydrate	8 g
Fat	0 g
Saturated fat	0 g
Dietary Fiber	4 g
Cholesterol	0 mg
Sodium	163 mg
Vitamin A	3 IU
Vitamin C	1 mg
Iron	1.5 mg

INSTRUCTIONS: In a small bowl, mix honey, soy sauce, sesame oil, and ginger. In large bowl, mix rice with sesame seed and then add the marinade. Add the crushed black seaweed (reserving a small amount to use as garnish). Form 1-inch balls. Place on a platter and sprinkle lightly with crushed black seaweed. You can also serve as a rice dish, without making the balls.

– From *"Common Edible Seaweeds in the Gulf of Alaska", by Dolly Garza*

139

Roasted Seaweed Popcorn

INGREDIENTS:

Black seaweed

INSTRUCTIONS: Fill a shallow pan with a single layer of black seaweed. Roast in an oven at around 175° F for 10 minutes. Check to see if it is roasted by trying to bend and snap a piece. If it snaps, it is ready to munch on like popcorn. Roasted seaweed may act as a laxative if you eat too much at once.

NUTRITION INFORMATION	
Per serving - 1 cup:	
Calories	40
Protein	4 g
Carbohydrate	6 g
Fat	0
Calories from Fat	6 %
Saturated fat	NT*
Dietary Fiber	5 g
Cholesterol	NT*
Sodium	150 mg
Vitamin A	632 IU
Vitamin C	2 mg
Iron	0.3 mg

*Not Tested

– From *"Common Edible Seaweeds in the Gulf of Alaska", by Dolly Garza*

Oven Roasted Kelp Chips

INGREDIENTS:

Kelp

INSTRUCTIONS: Roast kelp strips in an oven at 200° F for 5 to 10 minutes, or until seaweed turns green. Remove, cool, and eat.

NUTRITION INFORMATION	
Per 1 cup serving:	
Calories	42
Protein	3 g
Carbohydrate	8 g
Fat	0 g
Saturated fat	0 g
Dietary Fiber	4 g
Cholesterol	0 mg
Sodium	163 mg
Vitamin A	3 IU
Vitamin C	1 mg
Iron	1.5 mg

– From "Common Edible Seaweeds in the Gulf of Alaska", by Dolly Garza

Ribbon Seaweed Chips

INGREDIENTS:

Ribbon Seaweed

INSTRUCTIONS: Put some ribbon seaweed in a shallow pan and roast it at 125°-175° F for about 5 minutes. Remove from oven and allow to cool. It will crisp up as it cools. It has its own salt and flavor, so there is no need to add seasonings!

NUTRITION INFORMATION	
Per 1 cup serving:	
Calories	42
Protein	3 g
Carbohydrate	8 g
Fat	0 g
Saturated fat	0 g
Dietary Fiber	4 g
Cholesterol	0 mg
Sodium	163 mg
Vitamin A	3 IU
Vitamin C	1 mg
Iron	1.5 mg

– From "Common Edible Seaweeds in the Gulf of Alaska", by Dolly Garza

Beach Asparagus with Parmesan

INGREDIENTS:

2 cups beach asparagus, fresh or canned

2 tablespoons extra vigin olive oil

1/2 teaspoon lemon juice

1/2 cup parmesan, shredded

Black pepper, ground

NUTRITION INFORMATION	
Serves 4. Per serving:	
Calories	109.7
Protein	4.3 g
Carbohydrate	1.8 g
Fat	9.6 g
Saturated fat	2.7 g
Dietary Fiber	0.1 g*
Cholesterol	7.25 mg
Sodium	181.6 mg
Vitamin A	593.3 IU
Vitamin C	0.7 mg
Iron	0.5 mg

INSTRUCTIONS: If the asparagus is fresh, blanch for one minute in unsalted boiling water. If asparagus is canned, heat it in small pan for 5 minutes. Drain and place in a serving bowl. Make a dressing with olive oil and lemon juice, and spoon over the warm beach asparagus. Sprinkle with parmesan and ground black pepper. Serve warm.

– From "Common Edible Seaweeds in the Gulf of Alaska", by Dolly Garza

Akutaq (with seal oil)

INGREDIENTS:

6 cups berries

½ cup seal oil

½ cup shortening (Crisco)

1 cup sugar

NUTRITION INFORMATION	
Per 1/2 cup serving:	
Calories	296
Protein	2.2 g
Carbohydrate	27.5 g
Fat	21.6 g
Saturated fat	3.8 g
Dietary Fiber	
Cholesterol	7.9 mg
Sodium	1.2 mg
Vitamin A	852 IU
Vitamin C	136.6 mg
Iron	0.7 mg

INSTRUCTIONS: Mix the fat with the sugar. Add the berries.

– From "Alaska Native Nutrient Book", by Elizabeth Nobmann

Cranberry Nut Bread

INGREDIENTS:

2 cups flour

1 cup sugar

1 ½ teaspoons baking powder

½ teaspoon baking soda

½ teaspoon salt

¼ cup butter

¾ cup orange juice

1 tablespoon grated orange rind

1 egg, well beaten

½ cup chopped walnuts

1 ½ cup wild cranberries

NUTRITION INFORMATION	
Per serving - 1 slice:	
Calories	224
Protein	4 g
Carbohydrate	37 g
Fat	8 g
Calories from Fat	32 %
Saturated fat	3 g
Dietary Fiber	1 g
Cholesterol	24 mg
Sodium	182 mg
Vitamin A	161 IU
Vitamin C	16 mg
Iron	1.5 mg

INSTRUCTIONS: Mix together first five ingredients, cut in butter until mixture resembles coarse corn meal. Combine orange juice and rind with egg and pour into dry mixture. Mix just until damp, fold in nuts and berries.
Spoon into sprayed pan. Bake one hour at 350° F, or until bread springs back when lightly touched. Let set for five to ten minutes. Remove from pan to cool.

142

– Judi Christiansen, Seward

Berda's Blueberry Pudding

INGREDIENTS:

2 ½ cups fresh blueberries

¾ cup cold water

3 tablespoons all purpose flour

½ cup sugar

NUTRITION INFORMATION	
Per serving - 1/2 cup:	
Calories	83
Protein	1 g
Carbohydrate	21 g
Fat	0
Calories from Fat	0 %
Saturated fat	0
Dietary Fiber	1 g
Cholesterol	0
Sodium	1 mg
Vitamin A	0 IU
Vitamin C	7 mg
Iron	1 mg

INSTRUCTIONS: Whisk together cold water with 3 tablespoons of all purpose flour, set aside. Place blueberries in a medium size pot on med high heat, add enough water to nearly immerse the berries, add sugar and gently stir frequently as it comes to a rolling boil, it should start to thin out and become easier to stir. Add the water flour mixture. Stir frequently to prevent lumps, pudding should begin to thicken as it comes to a boil for up to 2 minutes. Cool completely and serve chilled or at room temperature.

Optional: serve with whipped cream or if too thick, add small amount of milk or canned milk.

143

Makes 8-10 servings

- Roberta Miljure, Anchorage (orginally from Aleknagik)

Alaska Salmon in Blanket

INGREDIENTS:

Alaska salmon fillets cut in eight 1" x 3" pieces (1 oz. each)

Canola oil spray (as needed)

Salt and pepper to taste

½ cup Honey barbeque sauce

1 eight oz. package of crescent rolls or
pizza dough

INSTRUCTIONS: Spray baking sheet with oil. Place Alaska salmon pieces on baking sheet and spray with oil. Season lightly with salt and pepper. Roast at 350° F for about 8 minutes. Set to cool.

NUTRITION INFORMATION	
Per serving - 3 oz.:	
Calories	207
Protein	9 g
Carbohydrate	31 g
Fat	4 g
Calories from Fat	19 %
Saturated fat	1 g
Dietary Fiber	1 g
Cholesterol	19 mg
Sodium	579 mg
Vitamin A	0 IU
Vitamin C	0 mg
Iron	1 mg

Unwrap rolls and spread out in triangles. Brush ½ teaspoon of honey barbeque sauce on each of the triangles. Place a strip of fish at the wide end of each triangle and roll up to enclose. Place point side down on the baking sheet. Bake at 350° F for 15 to 17 minutes. Serve with honey barbeque sauce or other prepared sauces.

144

– Alaska Seafood Marketing Institute Children's E-cookbook
  (www.wildalaskaflavor.com)

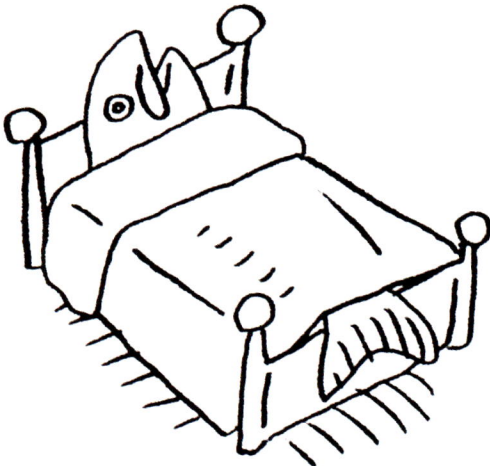

Crispy-crunchy Wild Alaska Pollock or Cod Fish Fingers

INGREDIENTS: :

1 pound wild Alaska pollock or cod fillet

1 to 2 tablespoons vegetable oil

1 large egg

½ cup breadcrumbs

3 tablespoons water

Salt and pepper to taste

NUTRITION INFORMATION	
Per serving - 1 oz:	
Calories	104
Protein	10 g
Carbohydrate	6 g
Fat	5 g
Calories from Fat	41 %
Saturated fat	1 g
Dietary Fiber	NT*
Cholesterol	52
Sodium	230 mg
Vitamin A	150 IU
Vitamin C	1 mg
Iron	0.54 mg

*Not Tested

INSTRUCTIONS: Preheat the oven to 400° F. Grease a baking sheet with a little vegetable oil. Cut the pollock or cod fillet into even-sized "fingers." Season them with a little salt and pepper. Beat the egg in a shallow dish with three tablespoons of cold water. Sprinkle the breadcrumbs onto a plate. Dip the fish fingers into the egg mixture, then roll them in the breadcrumbs and arrange on the baking sheet, allowing space between them. Bake for 15 to 20 minutes, until crisp and golden brown. While they are cooking, mix together the ingredients for the dip. Serve with dipping sauces and your choice of tasty vegetable.

145

Dip:

3 tablespoons mayonnaise

3 tablespoons ketchup

1 tablespoon finely chopped chives or onion

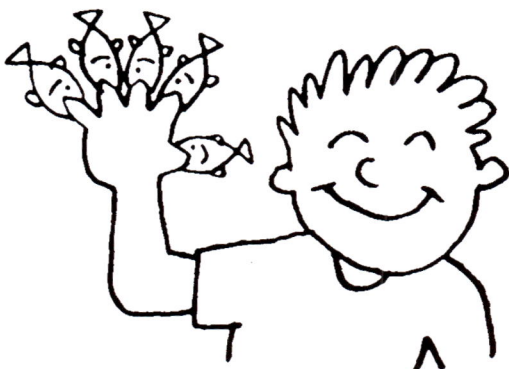

Blueberry Oatmeal Squares

INGREDIENTS:

1 ½ cups oatmeal

½ cup whole-wheat flour

½ teaspoon baking soda

½ teaspoon salt

1 teaspoon cinnamon

½ cup blueberries
(fresh or frozen)

1 egg

1 cup low-fat milk

3 tablespoons apple sauce

¼ cup brown sugar

NUTRITION INFORMATION	
Per serving - 1/2 cup:	
Calories	133
Protein	5 g
Carbohydrate	25 g
Fat	2 g
Calories from Fat	14 %
Saturated fat	1 g
Dietary Fiber	2 g
Cholesterol	22 mg
Sodium	250 mg
Vitamin A	100 IU
Vitamin C	2 mg
Iron	1.3 mg

146

INSTRUCTIONS: Have an adult preheat oven to 350 degrees F. Lightly coat a baking pan with cooking oil. Mix all ingredients together in a large bowl until combined. Pour into pan and bake for 20 minutes. Allow to cool for 5 minutes and cut into squares.

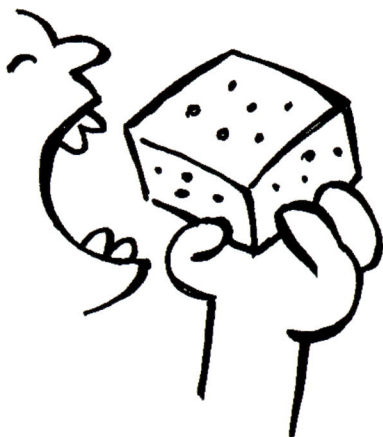

Pizza Pizzazz

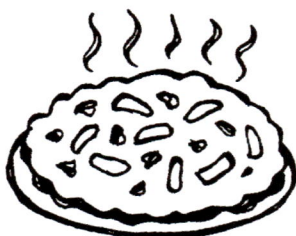

INGREDIENTS:

Pilot bread or bagel

Tomato sauce

Low-fat cheese

Your favorite vegetable

NUTRITION INFORMATION	
Per serving - 1 Pilot Bread	
Calories	153
Protein	8 g
Carbohydrate	23 g
Fat	3 g
Calories from Fat	15 %
Saturated fat	1 g
Dietary Fiber	2 g
Cholesterol	0
Sodium	669 mg
Vitamin A	500 IU
Vitamin C	4 mg
Iron	1.6 mg

INSTRUCTIONS: Top Pilot bread, ½ bagel
or ½ english muffin with tomato sauce, add small pieces of
vegetable and low-fat cheese. Have an adult warm up in oven
for you. Yum!

Juicy Pops

INGREDIENTS:

1 cup orange juice

small paper cups

1 cup apple juice

plastic spoons

1 cup berries

tin foil

NUTRITION INFORMATION	
Per serving - 6 oz:	
Calories	75
Protein	1 g
Carbohydrate	18 g
Fat	1 g
Calories from Fat	6 %
Saturated fat	0
Dietary Fiber	1 g
Cholesterol	0
Sodium	2 mg
Vitamin A	0 IU
Vitamin C	78 mg
Iron	0.9 mg

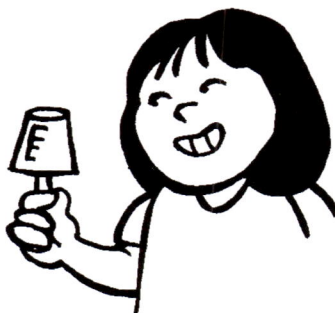

INSTRUCTIONS: Mix ingredients together,
pour into small paper cups, cover each cup with
tin foil, insert plastic spoon in cup, and freeze.
Once frozen , enjoy a cool treat by
peeling away paper cup!

Moose & Caribou Parts

Head The head is one of the best parts of a moose. Nearly all its tissues and meat are eaten, except for the glands which are not used from any animal. Head meat is very rich and is usually cut from the skull for cooking "moosehead soup" or "head cheese." Sometimes an entire head is suspended over a campfire and roasted—this is a great delicacy.

Nose This is boiled, roasted in a campfire, or dried and then soaked and boiled for eating.

Eyes Eyeballs are not eaten, but surrounding tissues and fat are boiled and eaten. Fat is also dried or eaten raw.

Ears Cartilage at the base of the ears is boiled or roasted for eating.

Tongue Often eaten after boiling, roasting or drying.

Lower jaw The entire jaw is boiled then the meat and tissues are eaten. Marrow from inside the jawbone is also eaten. The lower jaw is tabooed for all except old men.

Lips and mouth tissues Cooked and eaten but the lower lip is tabooed for all except old men. Tabooed parts are not included in dishes such as moosehead soup.

Head muscles are cooked and eaten.

Brain used in preparing "head cheese" and in tanning hides.

Neck All meat from the neck is eaten, except that from the first joint, which is permitted only to old people beyond childbearing age. Like most taboos on food, this one is imposed to prevent undesirable characteristics in the user's children. Often the penalty for eating tabooed foods is slowness or clumsiness.

Shoulder blade The shoulder meat is cooked or dried, and the moose's scapula can be dried and used for a moose call.

Foreleg The upper leg muscles and lower leg muscles are cooked and dried. The marrow is eaten raw or cooked. Joints of the leg bones may be pulverized and boiled to obtain grease. The lower foreleg bone is fashioned into a scraper for removing fat from animal skins.

Foot Forefeet and hind feet are boiled and the tissues are eaten. The feet are tabooed for all except old people.

Backbone The meat is cooked or dried and is considered very high in quality. This is especially true for the anterior meat along the high shoulder vertebrae. The bones are not used, but the spinal cord is removed from the cooked vertebrae and eaten. The sinew is removed, dried and used for sewing. Back sinew is considered the best for sewing and making snares.

Pelvis The meat is highly esteemed and is prepared by cooking or drying.

Tail This is cooked and eaten but is taboo for all except old people.

Hindleg The upper leg muscles are extremely valuable as food; the lower leg muscles are less preferred because they are too sinewy. The hind leg sinew can be used for sewing. The bones may be pulverized and boiled for grease, and the marrow is removed and eaten.

Ribs One of the best parts of moose or caribou. All rib meat is either dried or cooked, often for special events.

Brisket This is excellent meat, prepared by boiling.

Belly meat Dried, or boiled for a long period before eating. Considered a very good meat.

Lungs Sometimes cut into thin strips and boiled with meat; but primarily used for dog food.

Liver Cooked and eaten

Large stomach This is not eaten but may be filled with blood from the kill, frozen and then chopped up for dog food.

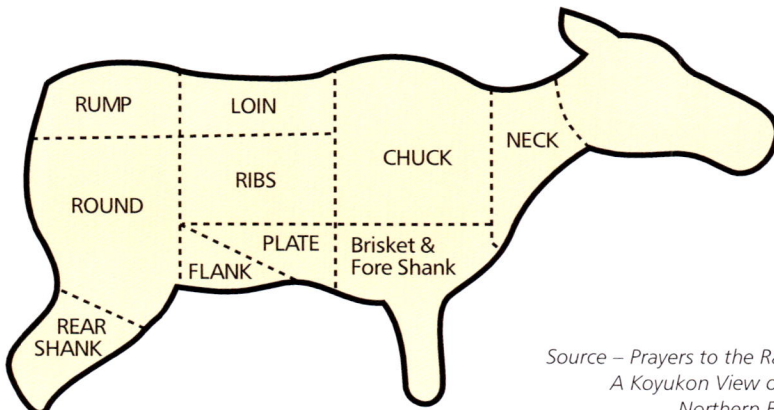

Source – Prayers to the Raven,
A Koyukon View of the
Northern Forest

NUTRIENT CONTENT & BENEFITS

Health Benefits Key: ♥ = heart friendly, ⬇S = low in sodium, ⬇F = low in fat, ⬇F = low in saturated fat, ⬇C = low in calorie,
⬆ = good source, 🏠 = great source, **P** = Protein, **I** = Iron, **A,C & D** = Vitamins A, D & C, **F** = Fiber, NT* = not tested

FOOD FROM THE LAND	HEALTH BENEFITS	Serving Size	Calories (kcal)	Protein (g)	CHO (g)	Fat (g)	Calories from Fat (%)	Saturated Fat (g)	Fiber (g)	Cholesterol (mg)	Sodium (mg)	Vitamin A (IU)	Vitamin C (mg)	Iron (mg)
Beaver - cooked	♥ ⬇S **P I**	3 oz	180	30	0	6	30%	2	0	99	50	0	3	9
Bone Marrow - cooked	NT*	1 oz	222	2	0	24	97%	NT*	NT*	NT*	NT*	68	NT*	1
Caribou - cooked	♥ ⬇S ⬇F **P I**	3 oz	142	25	0	4	25%	1	0	93	51	0	3	5
Deer - cooked	♥ ⬇S ⬇F **P I**	3 oz	134	26	0	3	20%	1	0	95	46	0	0	4
Reindeer - raw	♥ ⬇F **P I**	3 oz	107	19	0	3	25%	1	0	13	NT*	159	0	5
Hare (Arctic, Snowshoe, Rabbit) - cooked	♥ ⬇S ⬇F **P I**	3 oz	147	28	0	3	18%	1	0	105	38	0	0	4
Moose - cooked	♥ ⬇S ⬇F ⬇F **P I**	3 oz	114	25	0	1	8%	0	0	66	59	0	4	4
Musk Ox - cooked	♥ ⬇S ⬇F ⬇F **P I**	3 oz	122	24	0	2	15%	1	0	70	48	0	0	3
Muskrat - cooked	♥ ⬇S **P I**	3 oz	199	26	0	10	45%	NT*	0	103	81	0	6	6
Porcupine - cooked	♥ ⬇S **P I**	3 oz	217	25	0	12	50%	3	0	82	67	0	0	6
Squirrel - cooked	♥ ⬇S ⬇F **P I**	3 oz	147	26	0	4	24%	1	0	103	101	0	0	6
Bird Eggs (Sea Gull, Tern, Goose, Duck, Murre)	♥ ⬇S **P I A**	1 egg (duck)	130	9	1	10	69%	3	0	619	102	472	0	3
Black Brant - raw	♥ ⬇S **P I**	3 oz	151	28	1	4	24%	2	0	88	30	0	0	6
Canada Goose	♥ ⬇S **P I**	3 oz	139	19	0	6	39%	2	0	71	74	NT*	NT*	5
Crane (Sandhill) - raw	♥ ⬇S ⬇F **P I**	3 oz	135	29	0	2	13%	1	1	106	47	0	0	6
Duck - raw	♥ ⬇S **P I**	3 oz	105	17	0	4	34%	1	0	65	48	45	5	4
Ptarmagin - raw	♥ ⬇F ⬇F low cholesterol **P I A**	3 oz	109	21	0	2	16%	1	NT*	17	NT*	357	NT*	5

FOOD FROM THE SEA	HEALTH BENEFITS	Serving Size	Calories (kcal)	Protein (g)	CHO (g)	Fat (g)	Calories from Fat (%)	Saturated Fat (g)	Fiber (g)	Cholesterol (mg)	Sodium (mg)	Vitamin A (IU)	Vitamin C (mg)	Iron (mg)
Abalone (Northern & Pinto) - raw	♥ F S P I	3 oz	89	15	5	1	10%	0	0	72	256	6	2	3
Arctic Grayling	♥ S F S P	3 oz	79	17	0	1	11%	0	1	49	69	<100	1	1
Black Cod (Sablefish) - cooked	♥ S F S P	3 oz	89	20	0	1	10%	0	0	40	77	27	3	0
Blackfish - whole	♥ F P I A	3 oz	70	13	1	1	19%	NT*	NT*	NT*	NT*	1022	NT*	4
Clams - cooked	♥ S F S P I	3 oz	126	22	4	2	12%	0	NT*	57	95	145	1	24
Cockles (Heart Clam) - cooked	♥ F P I	3 oz	67	11	4	1	8%	NT*	NT*	NT*	NT*	NT*	NT*	14
Cod - cooked	♥ S F S P	3 oz	89	20	0	1	10%	0	0	40	77	27	3	0
Crab - cooked	♥ F S P	3 oz	82	16	0	1	11%	0	0	45	911	25	7	1
Eulachon (Ooligan, Hooligan, Smelt) - cooked	♥ S F P	3 oz	105	19	0	3	23%	0	0	76	65	49	0	1
Flounder - cooked	♥ S F S P	3 oz	100	21	0	1	9%	0	0	58	89	37	0	0
Gumboots (Leathery Chiton, Bidarkis)	♥ F P I A	3 oz	71	15	0	1	13%	NT*	NT*	NT*	NT*	1402	0	14
Halibut - cooked	♥ S F S P	3 oz	96	19	0	2	19%	0	0	64	73	136	NT*	0
Herring - cooked	♥ S P	3 oz	212	18	0	15	64%	4	0	84	81	99	0	1
Herring Eggs - raw	♥ S F S P	1/2 cup	63	8	4	2	29%	0	NT*	34	52	48	1	2
Hooligan Grease*	NT*	1 Tbl	135	0	0	15	100%	4	0	0	0	848	0	0
Lingcod	♥ S F S P	3 oz	71	15	0	1	8%	NT*	NT*	NT*	50	196	NT*	NT*
Octopus - cooked	♥ F S P I	3 oz	139	25	4	2	13%	0	0	82	391	255	7	8
Pike - cooked	♥ S F S P	3 oz	96	21	0	1	9%	0	0	42	42	69	3	1
Chum Salmon (Dog fish) - cooked	♥ S S P	3 oz	131	22	0	4	27%	1	0	81	54	97	0	1

*data based on Euchalon Grease

NUTRIENT CONTENT & BENEFITS

Health Benefits Key: ♥ = heart friendly, S = low in sodium, = low in fat, = low in saturated fat, = low in calorie, ⬆ = good source, 🏠 = great source, P = Protein, I = Iron, A, C & D = Vitamins A, D & C, F = Fiber, NT* = not tested

FOOD FROM THE SEA (continued)	HEALTH BENEFITS	Serving Size	Calories (kcal)	Protein (g)	CHO (g)	Fat (g)	Calories from Fat (%)	Saturated Fat (g)	Fiber (g)	Cholesterol (mg)	Sodium (mg)	Vitamin A (IU)	Vitamin C (mg)	Iron (mg)
King Salmon (Chinook) - kippered	P	3 oz	178	20	0	11	56%	2	0	57	740	35	0	0
Pink Salmon (Humpback) - dried	♥ S / P	3 oz	127	22	0	4	28%	1	0	57	73	116	0	1
Red Salmon (Sockeye) - canned	♥ / P I	3 oz	137	23	0	5	33%	1	0	59	332	184	0	2
Silver Salmon (Coho) - raw	♥ S / P	3 oz	123	19	1	5	37%	1	0	49	49	85	0	0
Salmon Eggs (Roe, Salmon Caviar) - raw	P	1/2 cup	212	25	2	12	51%	2	NT*	147	NT*	0	NT*	NT*
Sea Cucumber	♥ / P A	3 oz	58	11	3	0	0%	NT*	NT*	NT*	NT*	264	NT*	1
Sea Lion - meat with fat, raw	♥ S / P I A	3 oz	160	20	2	8	45%	2	0	53	61	246	<3	9
Seal - raw	♥ S / P I A	3 oz	121	24	0	3	22%	1	NT*	76	9	327	NT*	17
Seal Oil	♥ S A	1 Tbl	125	0	0	15	100%	2	0	NT*	0	487	0	0
Shrimp - cooked	♥ / P I	3 oz	84	18	0	1	11%	0	0	166	190	191	2	3
Sticklebacks (Needlefish)	P A	3 oz	86	8	1	5	52%	NT*	NT*	NT*	NT*	1046	0	5
Trout - cooked	♥ S / P	3 oz	128	19	0	5	35%	1	0	59	48	42	2	0
Walrus - raw	P I	3 oz	169	16	0	12	64%	2	NT*	68	NT*	144	NT*	8
Whitefish (Broad, Humpback, Pygmy, Round, Least Cisco, Bering Cisco, Arctic Cisco, Sheefish) - dried	P A	3 oz	315	53	0	11	31%	2	0	226	170	620	0	3
Whitefish Eggs - raw	♥ S / P C	1/2 cup	88	12	4	2	20%	0	0	373	136	257	10	5
Whale (Beluga, Bowhead) - cooked	♥ S / P I	3 oz	115	22	0	6	48%	1	0	24	85	280	6	12

NUTRIENT CONTENT & BENEFITS

PLANTS	HEALTH BENEFITS	Serving Size	Calories (kcal)	Protein (g)	CHO (g)	Fat (g)	Calories from Fat (%)	Saturated Fat (g)	Fiber (g)	Cholesterol (mg)	Sodium (mg)	Vitamin A (IU)	Vitamin C (mg)	Iron (mg)
Beach Asparagus (Sea Asparagus, Pickleweed) - raw	♥ S F C A	1 cup	15	1	2	0	0%	0	NT*	NT*	23	1057	1	0
Blueberry - raw	♥ S F C F	1 cup	88	2	18	1	11%	NT*	4	NT*	9	167	27	1
Cloudberry (Low Bush Salmonberry) - raw	♥ F A C	1 cup	76	4	13	1	14%	NT*	NT*	NT*	NT*	315	237	1
Low Bush Cranberry (Lingonberry) - raw	♥ F C	1 cup	82	1	18	1	8%	NT*	NT*	NT*	NT*	135	32	1
Crowberry (Blackberry, Mossberry) - raw	♥ S F F	1 cup	75	1	14	1	18%	NT*	5	NT*	4	67	7	0
Eskimo Potato - raw	P C	1 cup	202	9	34	4	18%	NT*	NT*	NT*	NT*	24	17	NT*
Fiddlehead Fern - raw	♥ S F A C F	1 cup	51	7	8	1	11%	NT*	6	0	2	5426	40	2
Fireweed (Wild Asparagus, Wild Herb) - raw	♥ S F A C F	1 cup	24	2	3	0	0%	NT*	3	NT*	28	3146	55	1
Goosetongue (Seaside Plantain) - cooked	♥ S F C I A C F	1 cup	25	2	4	1	29%	0	3	0	4	2026	33	3
Mouse Food (Mouse Caches) - Roots	♥ F C	1 cup	89	4	18	0	0%	NT*	NT*	NT*	NT*	NT*	18	NT*
Nettles Stinging Nettle, Burning Nettle, Indian Spinach	♥ S F A F	1 cup	37	2	7	0.1	2%	N/A	6	N/A	4	1790	N/A	1
High Bush Salmonberry (Salmonberry) - raw	♥ S F I A C	1 cup	68	1	15	0	0%	NT*	3	NT*	20	719	13	1
Seaweed (Kelp, Black, Ribbon) - dried	♥ F A F	1 cup	40	4	6	0	0%	0	5	NT*	145	613	2	1
Sea Lovage (Beach Lovage)	No Nutrition Information Available													
Sourdock (Arctic Dock, Sorrel) - young leaves	♥ F C A C	1 cup	34	2	5	1	14%	NT*	NT*	NT*	NT*	9520	54	1

NUTRIENT CONTENT & BENEFITS

Health Benefits Key: ♥ = heart friendly, ⌐S⌐ = low in sodium, ⌐☁⌐ = low in fat, ⌐☁⌐ = low in saturated fat, ⌐☁⌐ = low in calorie,
⬆ = good source, ⬆ = great source, **P** = Protein, **I** = Iron, **A,C & D** = Vitamins A, D & C, **F** = Fiber, NT* = not tested

PLANTS (continued)	HEALTH BENEFITS	Serving Size	Calories (kcal)	Protein (g)	CHO (g)	Fat (g)	Calories from Fat (%)	Saturated Fat (g)	Fiber (g)	Cholesterol (mg)	Sodium (mg)	Vitamin A (IU)	Vitamin C (mg)	Iron (mg)
Tundra Tea (Hudson Bay Tea, Labrador Tea, Eskimo Tea)	♥ ⌐☁⌐ ⌐☁⌐	1 oz tea	2	0	0	0	0%	0	NT*	0	313	0	1	0
Wild Celery (Indian Celery, Cow Parsnip) - cooked	♥ ⌐S⌐ ⌐☁⌐	1 cup	14	1	3	0	0%	0	1	0	68	87	5	0
Wild Rhubarb (Alaskan Rhubarb) - leaves	♥ ⌐☁⌐ A C	1 cup	49	3	8	0	0%	NT*	NT*	NT*	NT*	3584	26	NT*
Wild Rice (Chocolate Lily, Indian Rice, Kamchatka Lily, Riceroot)	♥ ⌐S⌐ ⌐☁⌐ F	1 cup	166	7	35	1	3%	0	3	0	5	5	0	1
Willow Leaves - young, chopped	♥ ⌐☁⌐ A C	1 cup	67	3	11	1	12%	NT*	NT*	NT*	NT*	10285	105	1
Stinkweed (Wormwood, Caribou Leaves, Alaskan Sage)	No Nutrition Information Available													

154

OTHER FOODS	HEALTH BENEFITS	Serving Size	Calories (kcal)	Protein (g)	CHO (g)	Fat (g)	Calories from Fat (%)	Saturated Fat (g)	Fiber (g)	Cholesterol (mg)	Sodium (mg)	Vitamin A (IU)	Vitamin C (mg)	Iron (mg)
Sailor Boy Pilot Bread (Pilot Boy Crackers)		25 g (1 piece)	100	2	18	3	20%	0	1	0	130	0	0	1

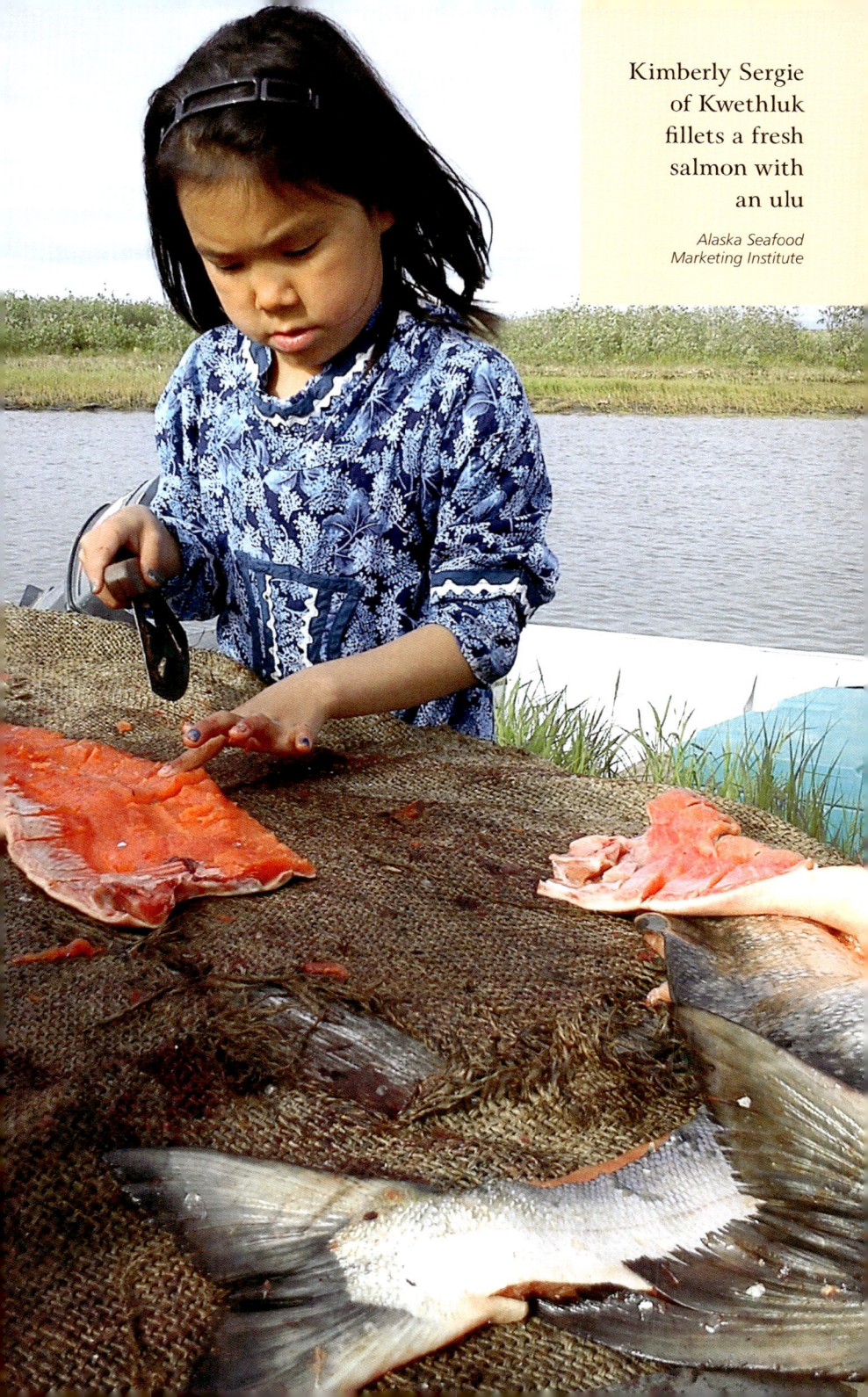

Kimberly Sergie
of Kwethluk
fillets a fresh
salmon with
an ulu

*Alaska Seafood
Marketing Institute*

FOOD SAFETY
Preventing Foodborne Illnesses

WHAT ARE FOODBORNE ILLNESSES? When infectious agents enter our food supply, such as harmful disease-causing bacteria, foodborne illnesses can develop. Individuals with a weakened immune system, including people being treated for cancer, are at higher risk for contracting foodborne illnesses.

> *"When the water gets warm, you can tell. The fish will spoil quickly"*
> – *Elder speaking about sheefish*

Signs and symptoms of foodborne illnesses are flu-like: nausea, vomiting, diarrhea, fever, headache and fatigue

COMMON CAUSES:

- Keeping dangerous foods (foods such as meat and fish that spoil easily) at temperatures between 45°F and 145°F for longer than four hours.
- Improper hand washing or cleaning of food preparation surfaces
- Contamination of one food by another, or cross-contamination
- Improper cooking methods
- Improper storing and freezing foods at unsafe temperatures

DO:

- Serve and consume cooked foods right away
- If cooked foods are not eaten right away keep them hot until they are eaten, or refrigerate or freeze them
- Wash hands before preparing food and before eating
- Wash food preparation surfaces before and after each use
- Use only clean utensils for eating, and transferring cooked foods to serving dishes
- Use two separate cutting boards: one for breads, fruits and vegetables, and another for raw meats, poultry, and seafood
- Wash fruits and vegetables even if you are going to peel them
- Clean the tops of cans before using a can opener

- Use food storage bags such as "freezer bags" to store food
- Store leftovers in shallow containers with covers
- Keep your refrigerator between 38-40° F
- Keep your freezer at 0° F
- Thaw foods in the refrigerator or microwave, do not leave food to thaw on the counter
- Cook all meats to an internal temperature of 160° F
- Reheat leftovers to an internal temperature greater than 165° F
- Throw away leftovers stored at room temperature longer than two hours
- Throw away leftovers older than two days
- Wash dishwashing cloths in hot water often
- Wash the top of soda and juice cans before opening. Pour into a clean cup to drink
- **BOIL FERMENTED FOODS BEFORE EATING THEM.** Although it may change the taste, boiling for 10 minutes can destroy the botulism toxin. This is important because you cannot see, taste or smell the botulism toxin.

DO NOT:

- Keep foods that spoil easily at room temperature – keep them hot or cold
- Refreeze foods once thawed
- Reuse marinating sauce on cooked foods, unless you boil it before using again
- Use utensils or plates that have come in contact with raw food
- Reuse food packaging or grocery bags for food storage
- Use garbage bags for food storage; they are chemically treated for garbage use only
- Use cutting boards for other foods after cutting meat or fish on them
- Put cooked food on a plate that held raw food

When in doubt, throw it out!

It is better to throw out food that may be contaminated than to eat it and get sick!

Food safety and environment

Alaska Native people live in one of the cleanest environments in the world with air, water, and food resources that support healthy lifestyles. However, our environment is not without problems. Important questions about contaminants and rates of cancer and other disease persist. There are also challenges related to monitoring and management of existing contaminants and global issues such as climate change and the Japanese Fukushima nuclear power plant accident that raise questions about emerging environmental concerns.

At this time, there is limited scientific data on contaminate related cancer incidence among Alaska Native people. There are areas of localized contamination including military and industrial sites where consumption of food and water resources is restricted. Additionally, Alaska Native people have unique exposures from contaminants that are deposited in the Arctic by air and water currents and concentrated in some traditional foods.

Studies to date clearly show that traditional diets are safe and that the benefits outweigh the risks. Alaska Native diet combined with an active traditional lifestyle is an effective approach to prevent cancer, heart disease, obesity and achieve overall wellness.

The connection between contaminants and cancer is complex and changing. ANTHC is actively involved in regional and community-level programs to monitoring contaminants and water and food safety. Consumption of traditional foods is strongly encouraged by the tribal health system for good nutrition, disease prevention and overall wellness.

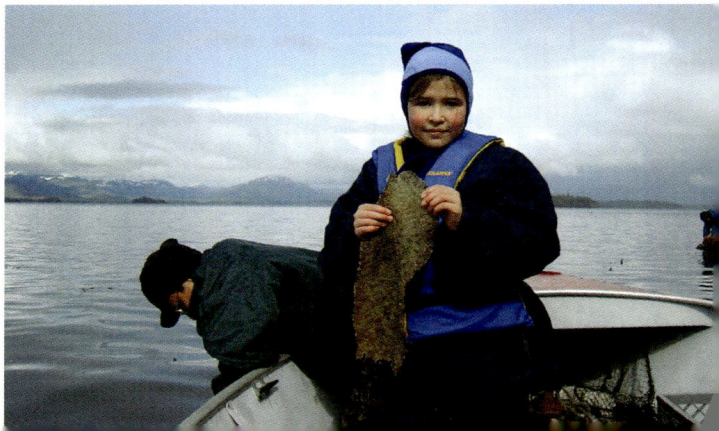

Herring eggs on macrocystis kelp.

George Nickerson

HAND WASHING

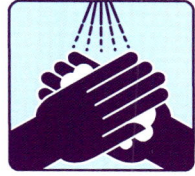

Washing your hands is a great way to lower your chances of getting sick —it also helps prevent the spread of germs and illnesses, such as the common cold, flu, meningitis, and Hepatitis A.

MAKE IT A HABIT! Hand washing steps to remember:

- Wet your hands with warm water (not cold or hot water).
- Apply plenty of soap and rub the front and back of your hands, wrists, between your fingers, and under your nails for at least 20 seconds. *How long is 20 seconds? A fun tip to help you remember is to sing a familiar childhood song like Twinkle, Twinkle Little Star, the ABC's or "Happy Birthday" twice, slowly.*
- Rinse your hands thoroughly with warm water.
- Completely dry your hands with a clean towel.
- Turn off the water with a paper towel when using a public restroom.

When soap and water are not available, use an alcohol-based gel or foam instant hand sanitizer (alcohol concentration between 60 & 95%). The 20 second rule still applies. Be sure to apply enough hand sanitizer (at least ½ teaspoon) to get your entire hand wet and rub your hands together until dry.

EXAMPLES OF WHEN TO WASH YOUR HANDS:

- When hands are visibly dirty
- Before, during, and after food preparation, especially after handling raw meat, poultry, and seafood
- Before and after being around sick family members and friends
- Before and after eating or taking medication
- Before inserting or taking out contact lenses
- After using the bathroom
- After changing a baby's diaper
- After being outside
- After sneezing, coughing, or using a handkerchief or tissue
- After touching computer keyboards and telephones in widely used areas
- After touching any part of the body, such as the face and hair
- After handling money, garbage, a pet or pet waste
- Any time you think your hands may be dirty

GLOSSARY

Appetite: Hunger or the desire to eat food.

Botulism: An illness caused by eating foods contaminated with a toxin, which can effect nerve function and have devastating affects on the body.

Calorie: A unit of measure, like gram or milligram, that represents the amount of energy our bodies get from food.

Carbohydrate: The main source of food energy for the body. There are two types: complex carbohydrates (which includes fiber) and simple sugars.

Cholesterol: An essential part of every cell in our bodies. It is made by the body and found in the some of the foods we eat.

Constipation: Bowel movements which are hard, dry and difficult to pass.

Cross-contamination: The spread of harmful bacteria from one food to another by direct contact or by dirty cooking utensils or hands.

Diarrhea: Runny, watery bowel movements.

Dietitian: A health professional with special training in nutrition, who can give advice on what and when to eat and answer questions about healthy eating.

Fat: The major storage form of energy in the body, fat is needed for good health.

Fatigue: Tiredness.

Fiber: A type of carbohydrate our bodies cannot fully digest, found in whole grains, vegetables, fruits and beans. It helps the body move the bowel to remove waste.

Foodborne illness: Any illness that results from eating food that is contaminated with bacteria or viruses.

Fortified: The addition of an essential vitamin or mineral to food to help meet dietary needs. An example is the addition of folic acid to flour.

Iron: A mineral used by the body to build muscle, to help the brain and body function, and to carry oxygen through the bloodstream.

Mineral: Found in food, a mineral is an essential element used by the body to maintain health and well-being. Calcium and iron are examples of minerals.

Nutrient: Substances in foods that provide nourishment to keep the body healthy and help it to grow. Vitamins and minerals are examples of nutrients.

Protein: An energy source in food made of amino acids. Proteins are used by the body to help cells grow and heal, as well as to build and maintain healthy tissues, muscles and organs.

Toxin: A poisonous substance made by other living cells or organisms that can have varying negative health effects when it comes in contact with the body.

Vitamin: Complex organic materials that play a key role in the body's health. Vitamins are found naturally in food. Supplements of vitamins and minerals are available in stores.

BIBLIOGRAPHY

Agency for Toxic Substances and Disease Registry (ATSDR). *What is Cancer?* Atlanta: ATSDR, (n.d.).

---. *Your Child's Environmental Health.* Atlanta: ATSDR, (n.d.).

Alaska Area Native Health Service (AANHS). *Dietary Intakes of Alaska Native Adults, 1987 – 1988.* Anchorage: AANHS, 1989.

---. *Taking Control of Your Body's Cholesterol.* Anchorage: AANHS, 1992.

Alaska Department of Fish and Game (ADF&G). "ADF&G Wildlife Notebook Series." http://www.adfg.state.ak.us/.

---. "Subsistence Technical Papers."

---. Alaska Fish & Wildlife News. "Stinging Nettle Tasty Table Fare." April 2006.

Alaska Department of Fish and Game (ADF&G), Division of Subsistence. "Subsistence in Alaska: A Year 2000 Update." http://www.subsistence.adfg.state.ak.us/

Alaska Native Health Board (ANHB). *Final Report on the Alaska Traditional Diet Survey.* Anchorage: ANHB, 2004.

Alaska Native Heritage Center. http://www.alaskanative.net/.

Alaska Native Knowledge Network. "Nutritive Value of Subsistence Foods Consumed in Alaska." http://www.ankn.uaf.edu/.

---. "The Positive Health Effects of Consuming Subsistence Foods in Alaska."

Alaska Native Tribal Health Consortium and Chugachmiut. Take the Idita-Health Challenge! 2008 Calendar.

Alaska Seafood Marketing Institute. http://www.alaskaseafood.org/.

Alaska Traditional Knowledge and Native Foods Database. http://www.nativeknowledge.org/start.htm.

American Cancer Society. "What About Sore Mouth, Gums and Throat Problems?" http://www.cancer.org/.

---. *ACS Guide to Complementary and Alternative Cancer Methods.* United States: ACS, 2000.

American Diabetes Association. *A Four Star Plan.* http://www.diabetes.org.

American Institute for Cancer Research (AICR). *Diet, Nutrition and Cancers of the Colon and Rectum.* Washington, DC: AICR, 2000.

---. *Diet and Health Recommendations for Cancer Prevention.* 2001.

---. *Nutrition and the Cancer Survivor.* 2002.

---. *The New American Plate: Comfort Foods.* 2002.

---. *Nutrition of the Cancer Patient.* 2003.

---. *Moving Toward a Plant-Based Diet: Menus and Recipes for Cancer Prevention.* 2004.

---. *A Closer Look at Energy Balance.* 2005.

Andrews, Susan B. and John Creed. *Authentic Alaska: Voices of Its Native Writers.* United States: University of Nebraska Press, 1998.

Association of Alaska School Boards' Alaska Initiative for Community Engagement. Traditional Values of Alaska [poster]. 2005. www.alaskaice.org

Baffin, Inuvik, Keewatin and Kitikmeot Health Boards, in conjunction with the Community Health Programs, Department of Health and Social Services, GNWT. *Nutrition Fact Sheet Series.* 1996.

Balikci, Asen. *The Netsilik Eskimo.* Prospect Heights: Waveland Press, Inc., 1970.

Biggs, Carol R. *Wild Edible & Medicinal Plants: Alaska, Canada & Pacific Northwest Rainforest.* Vol. 1, 1999.

---. Vol. 2, 2001.

Bragg, Beth. Alaska Staple Is Safe: Rumors of Pilot Bread's Demise Are False. *Anchorage Daily News,* November 6, 2007.

Brown, Amy. *Understanding Food Principles and Preparation.* 2nd Edition. Belmont: Thomson Wadsworth, 2004.

By Alaskans. *Cooking Alaskan.* United States: Alaska Northwest Books, 1990.

Centers for Disease Control and Prevention. "An Ounce of Prevention Keeps the Germs Away." http://www.cdc.gov/.

---. "What is Botulism?"

Centre for Indigenous Peoples' Nutrition and Environment, McGill University. "Traditional Food. A Good Source of Iron." http://www.mcgill.ca/cine/.

---. "All Fats Aren't Created Equal."

---. "Thinking About Traditional Food."

---. "Strong Teeth and Bones"

---. "Traditional Foods – Lean Meat and Fish."

---. "Vitamin A for Good Night Vision"

---. "Zinc for Healing."

Chandonnet, Ann. *The Alaska Heritage Seafood Cookbook.* United States: Graphic Arts Center Publishing Company, 1995.

Duncan, Pauline. *Tlingit Recipes of Today and Long Ago.* Lenexa: Cookbook Publishers, Inc., 2006

Dyer, Diana. *A Dietitian's Cancer Story: Information and Inspiration for Recovery and Healing.* Ann Arbor: Swan Press, 2002.

Easter Seal Society for Alaska. *Out of Alaska's Kitchens*. 1st Edition. 1952.

eHOW.com. "How to Make Hand Washing Fun for Kids." http://www.ehow.com.

Ellis, Eleanor. *Northern Cookbook*. Edmonton: Hurtig Publishers, 1979.

Ferman, Patricia. *Eat for a Healthy Heart!* Bristol Bay Area Health Corporation, 2002

Fienup-Riordan, Ann. *Eskimo Essays*. United States: Rutgers University Press, 1990.

---. *Boundaries and Passages: Rule and Ritual In Yup'ik Eskimo Oral Tradition*. United States: University of Oklahoma Press, 1994.

---. *Hunting Tradition in a Changing World*. United States: Rutgers University Press, 2000.

---. *Yuungnaqpiallerput: The Way We Genuinely Live, Masterworks of Yup'ik Science and Survival*. Seattle: University of Washington Press, 2007.

Foodconsumer.org. "Diet Before Cancer Treatment." http://www.foodconsumer.org.

Garibaldi, Ann. *Medicinal Flora of the Alaska Natives*. Anchorage: Alaska Natural Heritage Program, Environment and Natural Resources Institute, University of Alaska Anchorage, 1999.

Garza, Dolly. *Common Edible Seaweeds in the Gulf of Alaska*. Fairbanks: Alaska Sea Grant College Program, University of Alaska Fairbanks, 2005.

Golodoff, Suzi. *Wildflowers of Unalaska Island: A Guide to the Flowering Plants of an Aleutian Island*. Fairbanks: University of Alaska Press, 2003.

Graham, Frances Kelso and the Ouzinkie Botanical Society. *Plantlore of an Alaskan Island*. Anchorage: Alaska Northwest Publishing Company, 1985.

Halliday, Jan. *Native Peoples of Alaska*. Seattle: Sasquatch Books, 1998.

Hawai'i Department of Health, Healthy Hawai'i Initiative. *Eating by Color*. Honolulu: Hawai'i Department of Health, 2003.

Hawai'i Department of Health, Nutrition Branch. *5 A Day the Hawai'i Way*. Honolulu: Hawai'i Department of Health, 1997.

Institute of Medicine. *From Cancer Patient to Cancer Survivor: Lost in Transition*. Washington, DC: National Academies Press, 2006.

Jones, Anore. *Nauriat Niginaqtuat: Plants That We Eat*. Kotzebue: Maniilaq Association, 1983

---. "Iqaluich Niginaqtuat: Fish That We Eat." U.S. Fish and Wildlife Service Report. http://alaska.fws.gov.

Kari, Priscilla Russell. *Tanaina Plantlore Dena'ina Kiet'una: An Ethnobotany of Dena'ina Indians of Southcentral Alaska*. United States:

Alaska Native Language Center, Alaska Natural History Association, National Park Service, 1995.

Kavanagh, James. *The Nature of Alaska*. Waterford Press, 2005.

Krochmal, Arnold and Connie. *A Guide to the Medicinal Plans of the United States*. United States: The New York Times Book Co, 1973.

Lance Armstrong Foundation. Live**Strong** Survivor*Care* Program. www.laf.org

---. *Nutrition of Stinging Nettles*

Langdon, Steven J. *The Native People of Alaska*. Anchorage: Greatland Graphics, 1987.

Laraux, Sis. *The Alaskan Grub-Box*. Collierville: Fundcraft Publishing, (n.d.)

Mackenzie Regional Health Service and Keewatin Regional Health Board, Nutrition Program. *Nutrition Fact Sheet Series, Good Sources of Folacin*. 1995.

---. *Good Sources of Iron*.

---. *Good Sources of Vitamin A*.

---. *Good Sources of Vitamin C*.

Maniilaq Association. *Build Strong Families: Arctic Home Cooking*. 2nd Edition. Kotzebue: Maniilaq Association, (n.d.).

Mayo Clinic. *Disease-Fighting Foods: Smart Eating Choices*. Rochester: Mayo Foundation for Medical Education and Research, 2002.

---. "Handwashing: An Easy Way to Prevent Infection." http://www.mayoclinic.com.

---. *Your Guide to Vitamin & Mineral Supplements*. Rochester: Mayo Foundation for Medical Education and Research, 2005.

McElroy, Anne and Patricia K. Townsend. *Medical Anthropology in Ecological Perspective*. 4th Edition. Boulder: Westview Press, 2004.

Metcalfe, Peter M. *Gumboot Determination: The Story of the SouthEast Alaska Regional Health Corporation (SEARHC)*. Juneau: SEARHC, 2005.

Minister of National Health and Welfare, Health Canada. *Native Foods and Nutrition*. 1995.

Mitchell, Mary. *Nutrition Across the Life Span*. 2nd Edition. Philadelphia: Saunders, 2003.

Nail, Lillian M. "Strategies for Preventing Infection in Cancer Patients with Neutropenia." Oncology Nursing Society Congress, April 23 – 27, 2007. http://professional.cancerconsultants.com/

Nelson, Richard K. *Make Prayers to the Raven: A Koyukon View of the Northern Forest*. Chicago: University of Chicago Press, 1983.

Nobmann, Elizabeth. *Nutrient Value of Alaska Native Foods*. Anchorage: Alaska Area Native Health Service, Department of Health and Human Services, Indian Health Services, 1993.

Northwest Territories, Health and Social Services. *Northwest Territories Food Guide.* 2005.

NYTimes.com. "Hand Sanitizers, Good or Bad." http://www.nytimes.com.

Produce for Better Health Foundation. *5 a Day the Color Way.* 2005.

Schofield, Janice J. *Alaska's Wild Plants: A Guide to Alaska's Edible Harvest.* Portland: Alaska Northwest Books, 2004.

Schwartz, Anna L. *Cancer Fitness: Exercise Programs for Cancer Patients and Survivors.* New York: Simon & Schuster, 2004.

Selle, Mariko. *Traditional Food Access for Alaska Native Elders in Anchorage Long Term Care Facilities.* College of Health and Social Welfare, University of Alaska Anchorage, 2006.

Silver, Julie K. *After Cancer Treatment: Heal Faster, Better, Stronger.* Baltimore: Johns Hopkins University Press, 2006.

SouthEast Alaska Regional Health Consortium (SEARHC), Diabetes Prevention Program. Your Visual Guide to Healthier Eating [placemat]. (n.d.)

State of Alaska, Department of Health & Social Services, Division of Public Health. *Alaska in Action: Statewide Physical Activity and Nutrition Plan.* State of Alaska, 2005.

Sullivan, Robert J. *The Ten'a Food Quest.* Washington, DC: Catholic University of America Press, 1942*b*.

The Cancer Project. *Eating Right for Cancer Survival.* Washington, DC: The Cancer Project, 2005.

---. *Healthy Eating for Life,* 2004.

---. *The Nutrition Rainbow,* (n.d.).

The Alaska Geographic Society. *Alaska Geographic: Alaska's Seward Peninsula.* Vol. 14, No. 3.

---. *Alaska Geographic: The Kuskokwim.* Vol. 15, No. 4.

---. *Alaska Geographic: Native Cultures in Alaska.* Vol. 23, No. 2.

---. *Alaska Geographic: The Bering Sea.* Vol. 26, No. 3.

---. *Alaska Geographic: Living Off the Land.* Vol. 27, No. 4.

The American Dietetic Association and the American Diabetes Association, Inc. Ethnic and Regional Food Practices: Alaska Native Food Practices, Customs and Holidays. United States: American Dietetic Association and the American Diabetes Association, Inc., 1993.

Tohono O'odham Community Action. *Tohono O'odham Culture Calendar.* 2005.

---. Tohono O'odham Community Action and Tohono O'odham Community College. *Community Attitudes Toward Traditional Tohono O'odham Foods.* 2002.

U.S. Department of Health and Human Services. "Dietary Guidelines for Americans, 2005." http://www.health.gov/dietaryguidelines/

U.S. Department of Health and Human Services, National Institute of Dental and Craniofacial Research. *Chemotherapy and Your Mouth.* 2002.

U.S. Department of Health and Human Services, National Institutes for Health, National Cancer Institute. *Eating Hints for Cancer Patients: Before, During & After Treatment.* 2006.

---. *Nutrition in Cancer Care (PDQ®) Patient Version.* http://www.cancer.gov.

---. *Helping Yourself During Chemotherapy: 4 Steps for Patients.* 2005.

---. *Chemotherapy and You: Support for People With Cancer.* 2007.

---. *Thinking About Complementary & Alternative Medicine: A Guide for People with Cancer.* 2005.

U.S. Food and Drug Administration. "Basics for Handling Food Safely." http://www.fsis.usda.gov.

University of Alaska Anchorage. Institute of Social and Economic Research. "Alaska Native Education." http://www.alaskool.org/.

---. "Alaska Native Language."

---. "Subsistence."

---. "Traditional Life."

---. "Literature."

University of Alaska Fairbanks. Cooperative Extension Service, and U.S.D.A Cooperating. *Wild Edible and Poisonous Plants of Alaska.* 1989.

University of Michigan Integrative Medicine. *Healing Foods Pyramid.* http://www.med.umich.edu/umim

Wolfe, Robert J. *Playing with Fish and Other Lessons from the North.* University of Arizona Press, 2006.

Yukon-Kuskokwim Health Corporation (YKHC). *Native Foods: Treasures of the Tundra.* Bethel: YKHC, 1997.

---. Mary M. Gregory. *Yup'ik Native Nutrition.* 1991.

---. *Some Nutrients Found in the Food Guide Pyramid.* 1993.

ACKNOWLEDGEMENTS:

Alaska Native Tribal Health Consortium (ANTHC)
Alaska Native Elder Health Advisory Committee Members (ANEHAC):

Andrew Jimmie, *Chair, Minto*
Susie Akootchook, *Kaktovik* *
Rose Ambrose, *Huslia*
Ida Angasan, *Kaktovik*
Sophie Chase, *Anchorage* *
Anna Frank, *Minto*
Janet Guthrie, *Metlakatla* ‡
Rose Heyano, *Dillingham* ‡
Dan Karmun, *Nome* ‡
Ethul Lund, *Juneau* ‡

Iver Malutin, *Kodiak* *
Chris Merculief, *St. George*
John Morris, *Douglas*
Florence Pestrikoff, *Kodiak*
Mary Schaeffer, *Kotzebue*
James Segura, *Kenai*
James Sipary, *Toksook Bay*
Berda Willson, *Nome*
Lotha Wolf, *Mentasta Lake* ‡
Mike Zacharof, *St. Paul Island* *

Alaska Department of Fish and Game
  Groundfish Project
Alaska Fisheries Science Center, NOAA
  Fisheries Service
ANTHC Public Communications
Alaska Plant Materials Center
Alaska Seafood Marketing Institute
The Alaska SeaLife Center
Laura Apatiki
Audrey Armstrong
Carin Bailey
Eleanor Batchelder
Lincoln Bean
Rita Blumenstein
Kay Branch
Levi Brink
Scott Brylinsky
Patricia Bunyan
Vernita Bunyan
Alma Callis
Douglas Island Pink & Chum, Inc.
Irene S. Douthit
Gary Ferguson
Henry Frank
Dolly Garza
Marianne A. Gilmore
Robert Gorman
Joan Hastie
Judi Christiansen
Nina M. Heavener
Mellisa Heflin
Emily Hughes
Chuck Hunt*
Matthew Ione
Mike and Edna Jackson
Fritz Johnson
Anore Jones

Ruth Kalerak
Brenda King
Thomas C. Kline, Jr.
Harriet Kuhnlein
Francis Lampe*
Ann Lawrence
Richard J. Leland*
Rob MacDonald
Donna Malchoff
Eleanor McMullen
Millie McKeown
Roberta Miljure
Nora Nagaruk
Marilyn Neck
Natasha Nelson
George Nickerson
Patrick Norman
Fred Olin
Selma Oskolkoff-Simon
Andrew Pauken*
Martha Ray
Desirae Roehl
Frieda Seebold
Gloria Simeon
Quentin Simeon
Jeannette M. Smith
Tanana Chiefs Conference
U.S. Fish & Wildlife Service Alaska
  Image Library
Libby Watanabe
Tina Woods
Frank Wright
Donald Zanoff

* *Their wisdom continues to be shared
  after they have passed.*

‡ *Previous member*

"I go to Nome every summer and go to fish camp, go berry picking, and pick willow greens and sea lovage (tukkaayuk in Iñupiaq)... One of my favorite Native foods is fresh humpy soup with onion and tukkaayuks, served with seal oil... What I miss about living back home is going fishing for tomcod out at Nook. After the hole is chopped in the ice, you jig for just a bit, and pull out tomcod by the dozens. They insta-freeze, and we'd haul 'em home, slice them up with an ulu, and eat them frozen with seal oil." — Irene Douthit, Anchorage (originally from Nome)

"My mom, who is from Hooper Bay, hadn't been feeling well for awhile. She didn't have much of an appetite, and wasn't sleeping well. One day, a neighbor called to see if she wanted some cooked seal meat. She was so happy that they thought of her. She said she felt better after eating it — the seal meat "hit the spot," and helped her sleep better that night." — Karen Morgan, Anchorage

"When I was in the hospital, a lady from Nome was next to me and she wouldn't eat anything. They put food in her mouth, and she would turn her head away. Finally they told her IT'S A NATIVE FOOD and she opened her mouth and took the food."

- Elder

"My husband and son go out every summer, from May to October, in his home town on the lower Yukon and fish, and hunt moose and birds. So my freezer's full at home."

– Ann Lawrence, Anchorage (originally from Mountain Village)

"People used to be more active, and food was different. [We] need more information about healthy, organic food [Alaska berries and wild greens]."

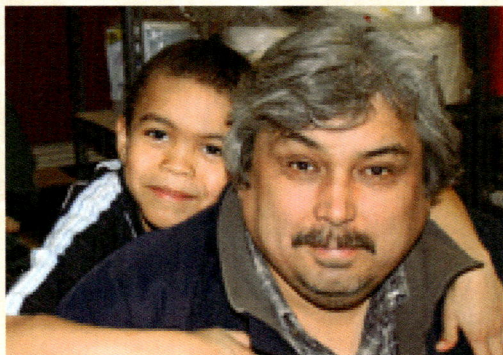

– Patrick Norman, Tribal Chief, Port Graham

Traditional Values of Alaska Native People

"Respect all living things" – Saint Lawrence Island Yup'ik

"Respect the animals you catch for food" – Cup'ik

"Have respect for our land and its resources at all times" "Share with others whenever possible" "Learn hunting and outdoor survival skills" – Bristol Bay Yup'ik

"Take care of the land" "Take care of the sea/ocean"
– Unangax (Aleut)

"Live with and respect the land, sea, and all nature" "Subsistence is sustenance for the life" – Unangan/Unangas

"Respect for land" "Respect for nature" "Practice of traditions" – Athabascan

"A subsistence lifestyle, respectful of and sustained by the natural world" "Stewardship of the animals, land, sky and waters" "Respect for self, others and our environment is inherent in all of these values" – Kodiak Alutiiq

"Respect for nature" "Hunter success"
– Northwest Arctic Iñupiaq

"Respect for nature – qiksriksrautiqaånia Iñuuniaåvigmun" "Hunting traditions - aÿuniallaniq"
– North Slope Iñupiaq

"Respect for nature and property" "We are stewards of the air, land, and sea" – Southeast tribal values

Select values are from the Association of Alaska School Boards' Alaska Initiative for Community Engagement Traditional Values of Alaska poster: